HAVE YOU EXPERIENCED THESE SYMPTOMS EVERY DAY FOR TWO WEEKS OR MORE?

- Changes in appetite
- Changes in weight
- Trouble sleeping or sleep disturbances
- Decreased energy
- Feelings of guilt, worthlessness, or hopelessness
- Trouble concentrating or thinking clearly
- Suicidal thoughts
- Slowed movement of the body
- Depressed mood
- Loss of interest or pleasure in activities you used to enjoy

If you answered "yes" to at least four of the above, you could be depressed and should see a physician for further testing and diagnosis.

ZOLOFT, PAXIL, LUVOX
AND
PROZAC

**All New Information to Help You
Choose the Right Antidepressant**

DONALD L. SULLIVAN, R. Ph., Ph.D.
Introduction by Craig Williams, M.D.

AN AVON BOOK

The ideas, procedures, and suggestions in this book are intended to supplement, not replace, the medical advice of a trained medical professional. All matters regarding your health require medical supervision. Consult your physician before adopting the suggestions in this book, as well as about any condition that may require diagnosis or medical attention. The author and publisher disclaim any liability arising directly or indirectly from the use of this book.

AVON BOOKS, INC.
1350 Avenue of the Americas
New York, New York 10019

Copyright © 1999 by Donald L. Sullivan
Published by arrangement with the author
Library of Congress Catalog Card Number: 98-91016
ISBN: 0-380-79518-3
www.avonbooks.com/wholecare

First Wholecare Printing: April 1999

AVON WHOLECARE TRADEMARK REG. U.S. PAT. OFF. AND IN OTHER COUNTRIES, MARCA REGISTRADA, HECHO EN U.S.A.

Printed in the U.S.A.

WCD   10   9   8   7   6   5   4   3   2

To my parents, Jan and Donna Sullivan; my loving wife, Amy; and my brother Jerry Sullivan, for all the love and support you gave me in writing this book. I will never forget all you have done for me. I could not have accomplished writing this book without you.

Acknowledgments

I would like to thank my family for all their love and support while writing this book. I would like to thank one person in particular—my wife, Amy—for all her help. She spent hundreds of hours editing my work, working on the computer, and doing many other little things that were greatly appreciated. I would like to thank my mother, Donna Sullivan, for all her work regarding pricing issues and verification. I would also like to thank my agent, Rick Balkin, for his hard work. His guidance and knowledge in the world of publishing are worth more than words can describe. I also appreciate all the hard work Dr. Craig Williams did in writing the introduction for this book. Finally, I would like to thank the publisher, Avon Books, for seeing the potential this book could achieve.

Contents

✎

Introduction

by Dr. Craig Williams, M.D.,
Director of Residency Training
in Adolescent Psychiatry,
The Ohio State University

Prozac, Zoloft, Paxil, and Luvox are such popular medications in the United States and abroad that we often hear them mentioned in conversation or see them advertised. Many of us know someone who has taken one of them.

These drugs are prescribed for many different conditions, including anxiety, depression, obsessive-compulsive disorder, and eating disorders, and current studies are looking at other potential uses. This book provides information about these commonly prescribed medicines. Because it does not consider the conditions for which they are prescribed, it does not make specific treatment recommendations. Neither should readers assume that these are the only medications that may be useful to patients. In addition, options other than medication may be helpful or necessary, given clinical conditions. The decision to start or stop taking medicine is best made in collaboration with a person's treating physician. Being more informed about the medications discussed in this book may help individuals to communicate better with their doctors if consideration is being given to prescribing one of them.

Prozac, Zoloft, Paxil, and Luvox have an effect on the serotonin levels of the central nervous system. Serotonin is a very important chemical in the brain, called a neurotransmitter, that is implicated in various disorders, including anxiety, depression, pain, obesity, nausea, migraine, obsessive-compulsive disorder, and stroke. Prozac, Zoloft, Paxil, and Luvox are members of the group of medicines often referred to as selective serotonin reuptake inhibitors (SSRIs). Essentially, they help the central nervous system make the most of the available serotonin within it by keeping the serotonin from being "reabsorbed" or "siphoned off" before it can be fully utilized. In the few years—less than ten—that these medicines have been available in the United States, they have become extremely popular.

Time and patience are often required before the most effective dose is found. Sometimes the initial prescription works well, but for many people this isn't the case. In addition, SSRIs do not take effect immediately. It may be weeks before patients experience any relief. Often the initial dosage needs to be increased, and the potential for side effects also increases.

But in fact, large numbers of people report having no troublesome side effects from SSRIs. Those who do may experience very mild ones and decide that they are worth enduring if the medicine has helped substantially. Some people report that the side effects disappear after the first few weeks. Others feel worse for the first few days after starting to take one of these medicines, and then begin to feel better. There are those, however, who cannot tolerate the side effects and need a change of medication. Interestingly, although all of the SSRIs have similar potential side effects, someone might experience a particular one while taking Prozac, for example, but would not necessarily experience it after switching to Zoloft. On the other hand, a side effect may remain the same or worsen when the patient tries a different SSRI.

Side effects include nausea, dizziness, drowsiness, and insomnia, as well as a variety of sexual disturbances. Although it may not technically be considered a side effect, some people suffer a "discontinuation syndrome" if they forget to take a dose or stop taking it altogether. This syndrome can involve a number of symptoms: fatigue, nausea, vomiting, dizziness, headache, irritability, and bad dreams.

Since the effectiveness, side effects, and price of these medicines are similar, how does one decide which one to take? Individual doctors may have different strategies for making this decision. These strategies tend to be based on the physician's experiences (both positive and negative) with the medications, as well as knowledge about them. Though doctors have multiple sources of information from which they can develop a knowledge base, sometimes little research or medical literature is available about specific or unusual topics. For example, the available hard data about the effects of SSRIs on children are quite limited. Pharmaceutical companies did few or no studies on the younger population when preparing to market SSRIs.

While information is now slowly becoming available about this and other special topics, such as the use of Prozac in pregnancy, there is still much to learn about these medicines. Thus a knowledgeable and experienced physician must match the patient's history to current options. Furthermore, the options may be influenced by certain guidelines and restrictions if the patient is in managed health care.

When I am evaluating someone for medication, certain information can be very helpful in deciding which drug to prescribe. First, it must be clear that the patient experiences symptoms that interfere with his or her ability to function. It is useful to know whether other family members have had similar problems and what their experiences have been with medications. I also need to know if the patient is taking other medications. For example, Luvox should not be taken with Seldane or Hismanal because of the potential for a very serious drug interaction. None of the four medicines discussed in this book should be prescribed for patients taking MAO inhibitors. In addition, a patient's general physical health is important. People who suffer from particular aches, pains, discomfort, or ailments may be at greater risk of experiencing side effects, some of which can be similar to the physical discomforts already present.

When I see a patient who hasn't previously been treated with an SSRI, I tend to recommend Prozac or Paxil first because it's easier to prescribe the right dosages effectively with these two medications.

If a patient has trouble falling asleep, I'm more likely to try Paxil first, because more of my patients have told me that they found relatively quick relief from insomnia when taking Paxil.

I explain to the patient that all medication has its limits, and that feelings of happiness may not result from taking it, though some of the depressed feelings will probably go away. After I prescribe an initial dose, I monitor the patient's progress and side effects in follow-up appointments. I increase the dose if the patient doesn't improve. If the patient experiences side effects, I must decide whether to change the medication or continue with the same course of treatment.

I do prescribe Luvox and Zoloft as well. Some people have a more robust response to these than to other SSRIs. Luvox usually requires a couple of doses per day, which some people may not consider convenient; finding the right dose may also take longer.

I have seen a variety of responses to SSRIs. One teenager told me that Prozac had changed his life. Indeed, he had improved in many ways. He was less irritable, seemed more energetic, and got more schoolwork done. But one day, his mother reported to me that the school had informed her that her son was falling asleep in class. Through a variety of errors, unbeknownst to me, his Prozac dose had been increased. Lab work showed that the level of another medicine he was taking had increased as well, probably as a result of the extra, unprescribed Prozac. When the dosage of Prozac was lowered back to the prescribed one, the problem at school was resolved. So it is important to continue to monitor drug levels.

Some patients develop a skin rash while taking Paxil. It is hard to know whether this is from the active ingredient, paroxetine, or from the substances used to compound it into a pill. Whatever the reasons, if you develop a rash switch to a different SSRI.

A mother once asked me to prescribe Luvox for her son, who had clear symptoms of obsessive-compulsive disorder. The youngster was already taking Prozac and had shown some improvement. His mother hoped a greater improvement would result if his medication were switched. When I spoke to the son, he confided that he had missed taking some of his doses of Prozac. I had to find a way to make the mother aware of the issue without betraying the boy's confidentiality. When that was resolved, and the boy's symptoms were reduced, his mother lost interest in changing his medication.

Though SSRIs help many people, I occasionally see patients who do not respond strongly to them. Fortunately, there are other classes of medication that can help them. The mind and body are enormously complicated, and as yet, those of us in clinical practice have no practical, precise way of measuring people's neurotransmitter activities. The serotonin system is not the only brain chemical system. There may well be brain chemicals that have yet to be discovered. Researchers continue to study the brain in order to develop options for those who have not found relief from their symptoms from among the current choices.

Practitioners must take into account many interesting variables. Practitioners and their individual patients must be able to agree on a course of treatment for each patient involving a scientific, individually tailored method to reduce symptoms and improve functioning.

It is my hope that the information in this book will prove useful to many people. Please remember that the use of these medications is a serious matter. Prozac, Zoloft, Paxil, and Luvox are not instant cures, and they may not help as much as we might wish. Nevertheless, they have been shown to be extremely valuable to people with a variety of conditions.

ONE

❧

How Do I Know if I Suffer from Depression and/or Obsessive-compulsive Disorder?

DEPRESSION

Christy is a twenty-eight year-old mother of one. Her child is well behaved and her husband is a dentist with a very successful practice. She knows her husband loves her, but he spends a lot of time taking care of his patients. For about the last month, Christy has not felt up to speed. She has lost interest in almost all the activities that used to provide her with so much pleasure, including aerobics, poetry, and ceramics. She used to enjoy romantic evenings with her husband that culminated in passionate lovemaking. Now, she can't remember the last time she even thought about sex with her husband. When he wants to have sex, she always makes some excuse. Christy has also noticed that she never feels like she gets a good night's sleep anymore. Many nights she tosses and turns for two hours before falling asleep. She always seems to be tired. Her appetite has also decreased substantially over the last month or so. Everything in Christy's life seems to be going well; she doesn't know why she's having these feelings or problems. Christy is most likely suffering from major depression.

People have been suffering from depression since the beginning of recorded time. Ancient civilizations wrote about depression as much as three thousand years ago. The ancient Greeks believed that depression was caused by excessive bile produced by the gallbladder. During the Middle Ages, scholars believed that depression was caused by God as an act of punishment and was not truly an illness. At that time, society felt depression was a result of the being weak-minded or full of sin. Even today, many misinformed individuals feel that depression is synonymous with "having a nervous breakdown." In fact, many great people have suffered from depression, including Abraham Lincoln, Ernest Hemingway, and Ludwig van Beethoven.

Many times the patient misdiagnoses depression. Everyone experiences days of feeling "down in the dumps." This is not the true definition of depression or of someone who is clinically depressed. The diagnosis, classification, and cause of depression are very complex. In fact, some physicians misdiagnose short-term or "down in the dumps" depression as clinical depression and use prescription drugs where they are not needed.

I've had patients come to my pharmacy and ask me if I think they are suffering from depression. They tell me they are feeling really "low." I ask them about their symptoms and I dig a little deeper into their problems. Many times things just seem to be going the wrong way for them or the patient is under a lot of stress at home or work. I explain to them that many people experience very similar feelings at some point during their lifetime. I also tell them that if their feelings persist for at least two weeks, they should see their doctor.

Data on exactly how many people suffer from depression are incomplete. It is believed that approximately

6 to 20 percent of the U.S. population may suffer from depression. Depression also seems to be more common in women than in men. In fact, depression in women occurs twice as often as in men. Even though depression can occur at any age, the highest rates of depression occur between the ages of twenty-five and forty-four.

Depression is also quite common in the elderly. It is believed that as many as 20 to 35 percent of the elderly who suffer from another chronic illness also suffer from depression. Genetics have been found to play a role in depression as well; depressive illnesses tend to occur within families. In fact, relatives of family members who suffer from depression are two to three times more likely to suffer from depression than others. The following discussion provides a brief overview of what causes clinical depression and how a patient can determine if he or she has it.

CAUSE

The cause of depression is too complex to be explained by only one factor or one theory. Life is filled with events that cause mental pain, including divorce, the death of a loved one, loss of a job, major illness, and more. Most people who face these challenges and/or changes and experience mild depression recover on their own and move on. However, some of these individuals may become stuck in a prolonged depressed mood.

The biogenic amine theory is one of the most widely accepted explanations of the cause of depression. This theory is that depression is caused by a reduction (decrease) of neurotransmitter chemicals in the brain. The decrease of these chemicals results in the faulty transmission of impulses within the central nervous system (CNS). In depression, this chemical deficiency is believed to be located within the limbic system. The limbic system is believed to control a number of important functions within the body, including sleep, appetite, energy, and motor functions. The decrease of neurotransmitters within this system creates a disruption of these functions and thus produces some of the symptoms of depression. This theory, however, doesn't totally explain the cause of depression. Other factors such as social and developmental factors may also contribute to causing depression.

DIAGNOSIS

The diagnosis of true depression versus normal grief caused by a situation such as the death of a loved one can be difficult because the symptoms may be the same. Grief is defined as a self-limiting reaction to a loss that requires no medical treatment. Grief can, however, become depression if the symptoms are severe and/or continue for several weeks. Suicidal thoughts, motor-function problems, and feelings of worthlessness are not common to a grief reaction. Such symptoms may indicate that you are depressed.

In my practice as a pharmacist, I've seen many patients taking antidepressants that should not have been. Some patients tell me they told their doctor they were feeling a little ''blue'' or ''down in the dumps'' and received a prescription for Prozac. *The blues are not depression.* All too often physicians use prescription drugs as a ''magic bullet.'' There is no true magic bullet for treating temporary melancholy feelings. These patients most likely do not need drug therapy. Patients who think they are suffering from depression should discuss this thoroughly with their doctor before taking any antidepressant.

The DSM-IV scale is the most common criteria used to diagnose depression. The major symptom of depression, using this scale, is a depressed mood or loss of interest or pleasure. This feeling is excessive and must be accompanied by other emotional, physical, or intellectual symptoms. These symptoms must be present nearly every day for two weeks in order to confirm the diagnosis of depression.

Sufferers experience a wide variety of emotional symptoms along with the depressed mood. Some of the emotional symptoms may include loss of interest in work or hobbies, change in personality, pessimistic feelings, crying spells, suicidal thoughts, anxiety, feeling you have let others down, feeling you are responsible for the sins of the world, hearing voices, and/or the belief that nothing will help you feel better.

Physical symptoms are also very common in a depressed person. Some of these include chronic fatigue, loss of energy, feeling unable to perform normal daily tasks, pain, headache, insomnia, early morning awakening, frequent nighttime awakening, decreased appetite, weight loss, heart palpitations, and loss of sexual interest. Conversely, some patients may experience the opposite of these symptoms, including increased appetite, weight gain, and increased sleep. Intellectual symptoms such as confusion, inability to make decisions, decreased ability to concentrate, sluggish thinking, and a poor memory of recent events are also prominent symptoms of depression. Finally, depressed patients may experience slowed physical movements and speech, agitation, and restlessness.

DEPRESSION QUIZ

This quiz is designed to help you assess whether or not you may be suffering from major depression. This quiz is not intended to replace the diagnosis of your condition by a qualified physician. Only a qualified physician can properly diagnose if you are suffering from major depression.

1. Do you have at least one of the following two symptoms?
   • I have experienced a depressed mood almost every day for the past two weeks.
   • I have experienced a loss of interest or pleasure in activities I used to enjoy.

If you answered yes to either question, continue on to section 2. If you answered no to both, most likely you are not suffering from major depression.

2. Which of the following symptoms have you experienced almost every day for the past two weeks? Check all that apply.
   __(a) changes in appetite
   __(b) changes in weight
   __(c) trouble sleeping or sleep disturbances
   __(d) decreased energy
   __(e) feelings of guilt, worthlessness, or hopelessness
   __(f) trouble concentrating or thinking clearly
   __(g) suicidal thoughts
   __(h) slowed body movement

If you checked off at least four of the above choices in section 2, you may be suffering from major depression and should see a physician for further testing and diagnosis.

It is important to know that not all patients experience all of these symptoms. Remember also that these symptoms must be present nearly every day for two weeks before the condition is truly diagnosed as depression.

The following chart provides a guideline for self-diagnosis of depression using the DSM-III-R.

DSM-IV DIAGNOSTIC CRITERIA FOR MAJOR DEPRESSIVE ILLNESS

A. At least five of the following symptoms have been present during the same two-week period and represent a change from previous functioning. At least one of the five symptoms must be either (1) depressed mood or (2) loss of interest or pleasure. One of these two symptoms is then accompanied by at least four other symptoms from the list below.
  1. depressed mood
  2. markedly diminished interest or pleasure in all or almost all activities
  3. significant weight loss (not from dieting) or weight gain, or significant decrease or increase in appetite
  4. insomnia, early morning awakening, increased sleep
  5. agitation, restlessness, slowed movement or speech
  6. fatigue or loss of energy
  7. feelings of worthlessness or excessive or inappropriate feelings of guilt
  8. diminished ability to think, concentrate, or unable to make a decision
  9. recurrent thoughts of death, recurrent suicidal intentions, or suicide intent or specific suicide plan

B. The mood disturbance is not due to an organic factor or is not a normal reaction to the death of a loved one or other very stressful situation.

C. The patient does not have delusions or hallucinations without prominent mood symptoms.

D. The patient does not have schizophrenia, schizophreniform, or a delusion disorder.

As you can see from this scale and the previous discussion of symptoms, depression is a very hard condition to diagnose. The DSM-IV scale is only a guide to the complete diagnosis of depression. When using this scale, the most important thing to remember is that at least five of these symptoms must be present nearly every day for two full weeks. If this is not the case, you are probably not suffering from clinical depression that warrants treatment. However, if you are, make an appointment with your doctor for a full physical checkup and discuss these symptoms in depth.

Talk to your doctor openly and discuss everything you are feeling. Ask your doctor if he or she feels comfortable diagnosing depression. Also, if your doctor does not ask you several questions about your depressive symptoms or give you some sort of depression assessment test, you probably weren't properly diagnosed. Very few physicians can properly diagnose major depression with only one or two simple questions.

The course of the illness is as variable as its diagnosis. Approximately 20 percent of patients will have only a single episode of depression in their lifetime compared to 80 percent, who will have some degree of relapse. The average number of depressive episodes in a lifetime, for those who do relapse, is usually five or six. Most treated episodes of depression last about three months, while untreated episodes last six to thirteen months. Many patients function well between episodes. However, about 20 to 35 percent of patients experience some degree of symptoms all of the time.

Depressive illnesses are not always so general. Specific types of depression have distinct characteristics. Melancholic-type depression, a severe form of depression, includes symptoms, such as mood swings based on the time of day (these are usually worse in the morning), early morning awakening, and significant weight loss. Seasonal depression, also known as seasonal affective disorder (SAD), is another common depressive illness. In seasonal depression, depressive episodes coincide with a particular sixty-day period of the year when symptoms occur. For example, patients may be depressed during the winter months, when there is less light.

Finally, depression should not be mistaken for dysthymia. Dysthymia is a chronic disturbance of mood involving either a depressed mood or loss of interest in most activities, but symptoms are not nearly as severe as a major depressive illness described under the DSM-III-R criteria. Dysthymia indicates a history of depressed mood more days than not for at least two years. Many patients with dysthymia mistake it for clinical or major depression. The diagnosis between dysthymia and major depression is difficult because many of the symptoms are the same.

Even though depression is often precipitated by some stressful or extremely emotional event, other diseases, medical conditions, and even some drugs may cause some symptoms of depression. Diseases such as cancer, endocrine disorders, thyroid disorders, lupus, chronic bronchitis, emphysema, cardiovascular disorders, multiple sclerosis, Alzheimer's disease, Parkinson's disease, some infections, and many others may produce depression-like symptoms. Substance abuse such as alcoholism and cocaine addiction may produce these symptoms as well. You should have a complete physical to rule out any of these conditions when you have the symptoms of depression.

Several prescription medications may produce depressive episodes or depression-like symptoms. These include: Aldomet, Amytal, Antabuse, Apresoline, Ativan, Butisol, Catapres, estrogens, Indocin, Ismelin, Lanoxin, Librium, Lozol, Minipress, Myambutol, Nembutal, Phenobarbital, Procanbid, Provera, Reserpine, Seconal, Serax, steroids, Symmetrel, Talacen, Tegretol, Tuinal, Valium, and Xanax, just to name a few. If you are experiencing some of the symptoms of depression, discuss your complete medical history, including current and past prescription medication use, with your doctor.

OBSESSIVE-COMPULSIVE DISORDER

Jack S. is a twenty-six year-old sales rep for a computer software company. He successfully rose from the mailroom to top salesperson in his region three of the past four years. His boss, colleagues, and customers all have a great relationship with him and he is highly regarded. Each morning Jack awakens at four thirty A.M. so that he can get ready for work. He has to be at work by nine o'clock. When he first gets up he heads straight for the shower. He spends at least forty-five minutes in the shower every morning making sure every inch of his body is clean. After he exits the shower, he spends the next forty-five minutes cleaning the bathroom each and every morning. He rubs vigorously at the bathroom fixtures until they shine like a new penny. While he's cleaning the bathroom, he constantly repeats to himself, "A thorough cleaning will prevent the spread of germs." Before leaving the spotless bathroom, Jack spends at least thirty minutes inspecting it, looking for areas he may have missed.

Then Jack gets dressed. He must count to thirty before each piece of clothing is put on. If Jack becomes interrupted or distracted by a noise, he gets completely undressed and starts all over again. Before he leaves the bedroom, Jack walks in and out of the bedroom doorway exactly ten times while holding his breath. Jack knows these practices don't make sense, but a feeling of anxiety overwhelms him if he doesn't complete these rituals. Jack suffers from obsessive-compulsive disorder.

Obsessive-compulsive disorder (OCD) is defined as recurrent obsessions or compulsions that are severe enough to be distressing, last at least one hour of every day, or significantly interfere with some aspect of normal functioning. To understand this definition, we must first define obsession and compulsion.

An obsession is an intrusive or recurring thought, image, or impulse that causes a great deal of anxiety. These thoughts or feelings cannot be ignored and are almost always on an individual's mind. Some of the most common obsessions are a feeling that everything is contaminated; collecting useless items; constant worry about whether a routine task was performed correctly; over-conscientious concerns about sacrilege, morality, or blasphemy; fear of not saying things exactly right; an excessive need to always have things in a certain order or arranged a certain way; and excessive superstitious fears. People with obsessions are preoccupied with these thoughts or feelings to the point that it interferes with normal activities of daily living.

Some examples of obsessive behaviors include saving ten years' worth of newspapers or old worn-out items; excessive urges to rape a family member or have sex with animals; fear of always hurting someone's feelings; and fear of starting a fire and burning down the house when lighting a simple candle. Many times these obsessions lead to a high degree of anxiety and nervousness.

A compulsion is a behavior or certain ritual an individual performs repetitively. This is done to reduce anxiety about an obsession or to prevent some future event from happening. Examples include the need to check the coffee pot or curling iron several times before leaving the house to make sure that they are turned off; counting money several times before paying someone; washing one's hands dozens of times a day to prevent contracting some disease; uncontrollable need to save mail, string, or wrapping paper; praying silently to neutralize bad thoughts; repetitive touching or the need for reassurance; and excessive cleaning, bathing, or brushing one's teeth. Most often it is adults, not children, who realize that at some point that their obsessions and compulsions are excessive and unreasonable.

It is important to recognize that everyone has day-to-day routines and some common fears. These routines help us keep order and structure in our lives. I've had patients who claim they're afraid of leaving the front door unlocked so they check it twice before leaving, or mothers who constantly check on their children playing in the backyard. Another patient of mine spends at least forty-five minutes in the morning getting dressed. She makes sure her hair, nails, makeup, and clothes appear almost perfect. This person works at a cosmetics counter, and her appearance is extremely important. These individuals are not obsessive-compulsive. Therefore, don't think that just because you are a particularly neat person or are very set in your ways that you suffer from OCD.

Individuals who do suffer from OCD take these routines, fears, and obsessions to very extreme levels. I had one patient who made her husband go back home at least twice every time they went out so she could check to make sure the stove was turned off. Once inside the house she checked the stove at least a dozen times. She was afraid of setting the house on fire. The husband finally took his wife to a psychiatrist. The psychiatrist found out about few of the wife's other bothersome rituals that the husband did not even know about. She was diagnosed as obsessive-compulsive.

OBSESSIVE-COMPULSIVE DISORDER QUIZ

This quiz is designed to help you assess whether or not you may be suffering from obsessive-compulsive disorder (OCD). This quiz is not intended to replace the diagnosis of your condition by a qualified physician. Only a qualified physician can properly diagnose if you are suffering from OCD.

If you answer yes to one or more of the following questions in parts I and II, you may be suffering from obsessive-compulsive disorder. These behaviors or rituals must occupy more than one hour of each day or significantly interfere with your daily routine or normal activities.

Part I (Obsessive Component)

1. Are you constantly concerned about contamination? Do you feel that everything you touch is contaminated with germs and may make you ill?
2. Do you become extremely distressed when things are not numbered or lined up correctly?
3. Do you collect worthless items like newspapers or an excessive amount of worn-out and useless clothes?
4. Are you constantly worried that some part of your body is not correct (example: one arm is longer than the other)?
5. Do you constantly worry that tasks you performed were not completed correctly?
6. Do you have constant thoughts of raping a family member or thoughts of having sex with an animal?
7. Are you excessively concerned about making God

mad at you or that everything you do may prevent you from going to heaven?

8. Do you have a constant fear of causing some terrible event like a house fire?

9. Do you always live in fear of saying the wrong thing and making someone mad at you?

Part II (Compulsive Component)

1. Do you excessively clean some household item(s)?

2. Do you wash your hands dozens of times a day or shower several times a day?

3. Do you find yourself always placing things in some sort of exact order or always arranging items in a specific fashion?

4. Do you find yourself repeating the same simple task over and over again such as opening and closing the refrigerator ten times before taking a can of soda out?

5. Do you have an uncontrollable need to save useless things like string, used wrapping paper, empty paper towel rolls, etc.?

6. Do you constantly check everything, such as opening the closet door ten to fifteen times to make sure you turned the light off?

7. Do you constantly confess everything for fear of telling a lie or getting into trouble?

8. Do you need constant reassurance from friends and family members that everything you do is correct?

Obsessive-compulsive disorder was once thought to be very rare, occurring in about 1 in 2,000 people. The consensus now is that OCD occurs in about 1 in 100 people. Men and women seem to be about equally affected, but men are more likely to be affected earlier in life. The average age when symptoms first appear is nineteen or twenty, but 33 to 50 percent of OCD sufferers first develop symptoms during their childhood or teenage years. One of the most distressing facts about OCD is that the course and severity of symptoms varies greatly between individuals and can be extremely unpredictable. In some individuals, the symptoms of OCD are very mild while in other people the symptoms are more severe and the individual suffers continuously throughout their entire lifetime. Symptoms often become worse during stressful situations and are often accompanied by depression.

Less is known about OCD than many other mental illnesses. The cause of the disease is believed to be similar to that of depression. For some unknown reason the brain and central nervous system have low levels of the neurotransmitter serotonin. Another explanation could also be that the system that regulates serotonin release is not functioning correctly. The exact role of serotonin in OCD is still not completely understood. As with depression, genetic factors are believed to play a role in those who are predisposed to developing OCD.

Dr. Craig Williams is a firm believer that the successful treatment of OCD is not only drug therapy, but psychotherapy as well. Patients must understand their obsessions and compulsions and identify how to modify these behaviors. Prescription drugs only aid in the ability of the patient to modify his or her ritualistic behaviors. Therefore, for someone with OCD, interaction with a psychiatrist or psychologist is very important.

If you think you may have some of these obsessions or compulsions, discuss them with your doctor. Treatment options are available that will help you gain control of your life again. The SSRIs (Prozac, Paxil, Luvox, and Zoloft) are becoming very effective tools in helping individuals overcome and cope with OCD.

However, you can contact a number of resources besides your family doctor regarding questions about OCD. Some of these are:

1. Obsessive-Compulsive Foundation, (203) 878-5669. This organization provides written information about medical referral services and counseling services.

2. Obsessive-Compulsive Anonymous (OCA), Box 215, New Hyde Park, NY 11040; (516) 741-4901. This organization provides a listing of OCA meetings throughout the United States and Canada. Publications regarding OCD are also available.

3. National Alliance for the Mentally Ill (NAMI), 200 North Glebe Road, Suite 1015, Arlington, VA 22203.

4. National Institute of Mental Health (NIHM), c/o Research on OCD, Building 10, Room 3D41, 10 Center Drive MSC 1264, Bethesda, MD 20892; (301) 496-3421.

T W O

❧

Prozac, Paxil, Zoloft, and Luvox:
A Breakthrough in
Treating Depression and
Obsessive-compulsive Disorder

Since the 1960s, physicians have believed that depression and OCD were caused by either a lack of neurotransmitter chemicals in the brain or that the system that regulates these neurotransmitters was not functioning correctly, causing the illnesses. The first breakthrough in the treatment of depression was the tricyclic antidepressants (TCAs). These drugs prevented the neurons in the brain from reabsorbing norepinephrine and to a lesser extent serotonin. When neurons send their messages in the brain they release the neurotransmitters norepinephrine and serotonin. Once the message is sent, these neurotransmitters are reabsorbed by the neuron to be used at another time for another message. This process of reabsorbing neurotransmitters is called reuptake. Remember, in depressed individuals there is a lack of the neurotransmitters norepinephrine and serotonin. So by inhibiting the reuptake of these neurotransmitters, more is available to send these messages. In the brain, these chemicals help us deal with stress, emotions, and so on. In the simplest terms, when the brain lacks these neurotransmitters, depression can occur. TCAs were developed first because these drugs affect only norepinephrine; serotonin reuptake in the brain had not yet been discovered.

The three primary neurotransmitter chemicals in the brain—serotonin, dopamine, and norepinephrine—send messages throughout the brain along millions of nerve fibers. The release of these neurotransmitters and their ability to stimulate neurons in the brain control everything from the ability to think and learn, our emotions, sexual behavior, coping with stress and hunger, and many bodily functions.

The monoamine hypothesis was one of the first theories scientists developed to explain depression. This hypothesis proposed that decreased concentrations of norepinephrine and serotonin at the nerve endings in the brain caused depression. Another theory developed by scientists, the norepinephrine theory, was based on the actions physicians observed when the drug reserpine was found in brain tissue. Reserpine was a medication used to control high blood pressure. This drug was also found to decrease the concentration of norepinephrine in the brain. Some patients taking this drug developed depression. Therefore, physicians concluded that the decrease in concentration of norepinephrine in the brain may be a cause of depression.

After further research, the norepinephrine theory developed into the permissive hypothesis. This theory emphasized the greater role of serotonin as a piece of the depression puzzle. This theory speculates that lower concentrations of serotonin in the brain, along with norepinephrine, cause depression. This theory, along with all the other theories before it, became the building block of the more modern theory called the dysregulation hypothesis. The dysregulation hypothesis is more complex than any of the earlier ones. This theory proposes that there is a disruption or disregulation of the system of neurotransmitters (norepinephrine and serotonin) in the brain. Either the brain does not have enough of these neurotransmitters or enzymes are breaking them down before they can exert their full effect.

Today, we realize that these "simple theories" do not fully explain what causes depression and OCD. In fact, very little is still known about what truly causes OCD and how brain chemistry is affected. Scientists and physicians do know that SSRIs help patients with OCD, but the exact mechanism by which they do so is still an unsolved mystery. However, from these findings and theories, it was determined that drugs that increase the concentrations of norepinephrine and serotonin in the brain have a significant effect in treating depression and OCD.

For years after their discovery, TCAs were the mainstay of treatment for depression and obsessive-compulsive disorder (OCD) along with some limited type of supportive therapy. These drugs included Anafranil, Asendin, Elavil, Ludiomil, Norpramin, Pamelor, Sinequan, Surmontil, Tofranil, and Vivactil. These drugs were effective in treating depression, but had a high incidence of unwanted side effects, including dry mouth, constipation, blurred vision, trouble urinating, and especially drowsiness, which many patients cannot tolerate. The drowsiness problem was somewhat overcome by giving these drugs at bedtime when appropriate, but other problems with TCAs soon materialized. I've had patients on TCAs come to the pharmacy complaining of a dry mouth so bad they feel like they could spit sand. Others have described the dry mouth caused by TCAs as "cotton mouth."

TCAs are also known for causing undesirable cardiovascular side effects such as fast heartbeat, irregular heartbeat, and quickened pulse. Some of Dr. Williams's patients on TCAs describe the fast heartbeat as "feeling like my heart is racing like a race horse." Others describe the cardiovascular side effects in the following terms: "it feels like my heart skips a beat," "my heart feels like it's beating funny," or "my heart feels like it's going to jump right out of my chest." These side effects may be harmful to individuals with various types of heart disease such as congestive heart failure, high blood pressure, angina, and irregular heartbeat.

Another potentially dangerous side effect of TCAs is postural hypotension, which is a sudden dramatic drop in blood pressure when rising from a sitting or lying-down position. Postural hypotension causes dizziness, unsteadiness, and lack of coordination for a short period of time, usually less than a minute. This condition is not life-threatening, but is very dangerous. The dizziness and unsteadiness associated with postural hypotension causes many patients to fall or stumble. This can lead to a number of injuries including broken arms, legs, hips, and so on. This condition is especially dangerous in the elderly, whose dizziness and unsteadiness seem to be more severe. Some patients who have experienced this side effect tell me when they get up in morning the entire room spins like a top.

TCAs can also cause an increase in the skin's sensitivity to sunlight, causing it to sunburn more easily. Although this is an uncommon side effect, I had one patient who learned the seriousness of it the hard way. The patient was in Florida on vacation and was taking a TCA. She went on a morning walking tour. She knew she would only be in the sun about two hours and the temperature was only 70 degrees, so she didn't bother applying a sunscreen. She ended up with a sunburn so bad she could hardly move. She could have easily avoided this by applying a sunscreen with an SPF of at least 30 half an hour before she went out in the sun.

Past research has demonstrated that these side effects are the main reasons patients quit taking TCAs for depression. In fact, some researchers suggest that 60 percent of the patients taking TCAs quit taking their medication due to unwanted side effects. Doctors were also finding that patients were taking lower-than-prescribed doses of TCAs to avoid the unwanted side effects. This problem leads to patients taking doses that are too low and produce limited or no benefit in treating depression. Dr. Williams has found that side effects are the main reason most people with depression and OCD quit taking their medication.

Two other major problems associated with taking TCAs were discovered over the years. First, it is relatively easy to overdose on TCAs in a suicide attempt. This is a huge concern with depressed patients who may have suicidal tendencies. TCAs are very toxic in high doses compared to some other antidepressants, particularly if combined with alcohol. Adding large amounts of alcohol to an attempted suicide with a TCA is like adding gasoline to a forest fire. Several deaths have occurred due to intentional overdose.

The other problem with TCAs is the seriousness of potential drug-to-drug interactions. The most significant interactions are those between TCAs and alcohol, anxiety medications, pain killers, muscle relaxers, antihistamines, and any other medication that has the potential to cause drowsiness. TCAs in combination with one or more of the above mentioned drugs can cause a significant increase in drowsiness and central nervous system (CNS) depression. This may result in confusion, low blood pressure, and respiratory depression, which can be deadly. Patients have told me that they feel like they were ''drugged'' when they combined a TCA with an allergy medication. A few have even passed out when combining a TCA with a strong pain killer.

Another dangerous drug interaction occurs between TCAs and sympathomimetics. Sympathomimetics, such as ephedrine, pseudoephedrine, and phenylpropanolamine are all decongestants most commonly found in over-the-counter cough and cold medications, allergy products, and diet drugs. The combination of TCAs and these products can cause very high blood pressure, fast heartbeat, and irregular heartbeat. TCAs may also affect the actions of some blood pressure medications and antipsychotic drugs as well.

There is no doubt that clinically, the tricyclic antidepressants are effective in treating depression. TCAs were by far the most popular drug used to treat depression before Prozac came on the market. In fact, the success of TCAs led to research into ways to improve upon their success and to reduce their side effects. The search for a more perfect antidepressant fueled research efforts that led to the discovery of the selective serotonin reuptake inhibitors (SSRIs) Prozac, Paxil, Zoloft, and Luvox.

The first SSRI, Prozac, became available in 1988. Almost overnight this drug enjoyed tremendous popularity with physicians due to its improvements over the traditional TCAs. It wasn't until the mid 1990s that three other SSRIs—Paxil, Zoloft, and Luvox—became available. Because SSRIs do not significantly affect norepinephrine reuptake or histamine receptors in the body, their side effect profiles are much better and safer. The drowsiness, constipation, urinary retention, and blurred vision occur less frequently in patients taking SSRIs. When these side effects do occur, they are less severe in nature.

You may think that drugs that cause fewer side effects are a terrific bonus, but that is not always the case. In Chapter 1, I made the statement that I've seen many patients on antidepressants that really shouldn't be on them. Because the SSRIs cause fewer side effects than other antidepressants, many physicians prescribe them for patients who may not need them. Some doctors may think that because the SSRIs are fairly safe, what can it hurt to prescribe them in a borderline case? It may actually help the patient. Patients must remember that drugs are chemicals and do have the potential to cause harm. Physicians should not let the safety of the SSRIs affect their decision regarding whether treatment is needed or not.

Dr. Williams, however, likes to use Paxil because of one of its side effects—drowsiness. Many depressed patients also suffer from some anxiety and insomnia. Paxil helps to calm their nerves and alleviate some of the insomnia. Over time, patients usually adjust to the drowsiness effects of Paxil and it doesn't bother them anymore.

Another improvement of SSRIs over TCAs is that patients don't experience postural hypotension, the short-lived drop in blood pressure after rising from a seated or prone position. Therefore, SSRIs are safer to use in the elderly, who are more prone to postural hypotension and the serious falls and injuries that it can cause. SSRIs also don't cause the nasty cardiac problems that TCAs may cause. This makes them safer to use in individuals with heart disease, heart failure, high blood pressure, and in patients who have irregular heartbeat. In fact, due to fewer side effects and a better safety profile, patients taking SSRIs are much more likely to continue with their treatment than patients taking TCAs.

However, one side effect that does tend to be particularly bothersome to patients taking SSRIs is sexual dysfunction. Decreased sex drive, difficulty or delay in having an orgasm, difficulty in ejaculating, and/or impotence may become problems. The manufacturers of the SSRIs reported in clinical testing that these problems occurred in a relatively small percentage of patients. After a few years and several million patients taking these drugs, doctors have seen the actual occurrence of sexual dysfunction to be significantly higher.

Because most patients don't discuss sexual side effects with their doctor or pharmacist, the true percentage of patients affected is unknown. Some physicians believe that as many as 70 percent of patients taking an SSRI may experience some form of sexual dysfunction, of which many are mild. In some patients, the problem may resolve itself after continued use of the drug. Some physicians have suggested using lower doses or skipping doses on Friday and Saturday as ways of decreasing the incidence and severity of sexual dysfunction side effects. It is worth mentioning that many medications can cause sexual dysfunction, including the TCAs. Any patient experiencing any type of sexual dysfunction should discuss this with his or her doctor and pharmacist.

Dr. Williams recalls one patient who was taking an antidepressant from the TCA family of drugs. This patient was switched to Prozac because of the higher potential for side effects and adverse drug reactions with TCAs as compared to SSRIs. After starting Prozac, the patient saw her sex drive decrease significantly and was unable to have an orgasm during sex with her husband. So that her husband wouldn't feel bad, she faked her orgasm every time they had sex. This became such a problem that after several months she had virtually no interest in sex. It was not pleasurable any more. She finally decided to take her chances with other side effects and convinced her doctor to switch her back to the TCA. I've had patients tell me they would rather take their chances with depression than give up sex. If patients would just discuss these sexual side effects with their doctor, he or she could try them on another antidepressant medication, with possibly better results.

Gastrointestinal (GI) side effects seem to be more common with SSRIs than TCAs. These side effects include nausea, gas, bloating, vomiting, and diarrhea. Nausea and diarrhea are by far the most common of all GI side effects. Many times these side effects are mild and disappear by themselves with continued use of an SSRI. I have found (and other doctors agree) that patients on Zoloft tend to experience more GI side effects, especially diarrhea and nausea, than with the other SSRIs. If you examine the clinical study results from Pfizer, the maker of the drug, Zoloft does have a slightly higher incidence of GI side effects.

SSRIs are definitively safer than TCAs in regard to drug-to-drug interactions, with a few exceptions. SSRIs cannot be taken with monoamine oxidase (MAO) inhibitors. This combination can cause what is known as serotonin syndrome, a condition that can range from very mild to deadly. The symptoms of serotonin syndrome are high blood pressure, high body temperature, fast heartbeat, confusion, extreme nervousness, delirious behavior, and even coma. This drug interaction is widely known by health-care professionals. It can be avoided by not taking Paxil, Zoloft, or Luvox within two weeks of taking Eldepryl, Furoxone, Nardil, or Parnate; avoid these drugs within five to six weeks of taking Prozac. For a complete discussion of the drug interactions for each SSRI, refer to chapters 3 through 6, which discuss each drug individually.

A big advantage of SSRIs over TCAs is in the lighter effect alcohol, anxiety medications, pain killers, muscle relaxers, antihistamines, and any other medication that has the potential to cause drowsiness have on the SSRIs. Such drugs do not cause nearly as much drowsiness, and respiratory depression when taken with SSRIs as compared to TCAs. SSRIs will, however, cause some limited drowsiness so caution should be used. Tolerance to this drowsiness usually develops over time.

Also, it is much more difficult to overdose in a suicide attempt with an SSRI than with TCAs. Patients would literally have to take dozens of extra doses of an SSRI all at once, and even then the risk of death is minimal. This makes the SSRIs safer to give to patients who may have suicidal tendencies. There has been a lot of press regarding the SSRIs, especially Prozac, "driving" patients to commit suicide. This accusation is completely unfounded and no sound scientific evidence has been presented to back it up. However, suicidal patients taking SSRIs should be monitored very carefully and be given only enough medication for small periods of time, if possible.

The above discussion has presented a brief description of how antidepressants work in the body and of the differences between TCAs and SSRIs. It must be noted that many physicians believe that SSRIs have not been found to be any more effective than TCAs. The advantages of SSRIs over TCAs that makes them the drug of choice are:

1. decreased incidence and severity of side effects
2. lower toxicity (meaning it is harder for patients to overdose on SSRIs versus TCAs)
3. decreased potential for severe drug interactions
4. better chance of patients complying with therapy and continuing treatment

Now that you have a basic understanding of the SSRIs and how they work, refer to each individual chapter dedicated to each individual SSRI.

THREE

❧

Luvox

BRAND NAME

The brand name of the drug is Luvox.

GENERIC NAME

The generic name of the drug is fluvoxamine. Currently no generic form is available. The patent on the drug expires sometime after the year 1999. By this time, a generic alternative may be available.

DOSAGE FORMS

Luvox is available in 25mg, 50mg, and 100mg tablets. The drug is currently not available in a liquid form.

APPROVED AND ACCEPTED USES

Luvox has not been approved for use in adult patients with major depression, but has been used to treat tens of thousands of patients with depression in the United States and worldwide. The drug has been approved to treat major depression in Europe and Canada; it was first approved for this use in Switzerland in 1983. Formal FDA approval to treat major depression in the United States should be forthcoming soon.

A major depression episode is defined as a persistent depressed mood that interferes with daily functioning nearly every day for at least two weeks. It should also include at least four of the following eight symptoms: change in appetite, change in sleep, loss of interest in usual activities, decreased sex drive, increased feeling of tiredness, feeling of guilt or worthlessness, slowed thinking or impaired concentration, and a suicide attempt or thoughts of suicide.

Luvox has been approved for use in obsessive-compulsive disorder (OCD). OCD is defined as the obsessions or compulsions that cause extreme distress, are time-consuming, or significantly interfere with functioning socially or at work. The patient recognizes these behaviors as excessive and unreasonable, but still cannot control the urge to perform them. A unique characteristic of Luvox is that it is the only drug in its class formally approved to treat OCD in children.

USUAL DOSE

The usual dose in treating depression is 100mg to 200mg per day. Most patients are started on a 50mg or 100mg dose at bedtime for the first week of treatment. In some patients, doses as high as 250mg or 300mg per day may be needed in order to obtain the desired antidepressive effect. Doses of Luvox may be increased to a maximum of 300mg per day by a physician after several weeks if no significant improvement of the symptoms is seen. The dosage of the drug may be increased in 50mg increments. Physicians should wait at least four to seven days between dosage increases. If the daily dose is more than 100mg, the dose should be equally divided in two. These

higher doses should be taken in the morning and at bedtime. If the daily dose cannot be equally divided, the
larger of the two doses should be taken at bedtime. Individuals should not take more than 300mg of Luvox
per day. The drug may require several weeks of treatment before patients feel noticeable improvement. Individuals should not expect immediate results or a
spontaneous miracle when taking the drug.

The usual adult dose for obsessive-compulsive disorder (OCD) is 100mg to 200mg once daily. Higher doses
of 200mg to 300mg per day may be used if, after several
weeks of treatment with lower doses, no improvement
is seen. Patients should be started on 50mg per day at
bedtime. Doses may be increased by 50mg every four to
seven days until the drug achieves the desired effect. If
the daily dose is more than 100mg, the dose should be
equally divided in two. These higher doses should be
taken in the morning and at bedtime. If the daily dose
cannot be equally divided, the larger of the two doses
should be taken at bedtime. As with depression, individuals should not take more than 300mg of Luvox per day
for OCD. Doses for children with OCD are discussed in
the section "Use in Children."

ONSET OF ACTIVITY AND LENGTH
OF ACTION

After a single dose of Luvox has been taken, the drug
stays in the body for approximately sixteen hours. After
several days of use, the drug stays in the body approximately thirty-two hours. It usually takes between two to
four weeks before patients see noticeable improvement
in symptoms. In some individuals the time period for
improvement may be several weeks or even a few
months. If the patient sees no improvement after several
weeks, the physician may want to consider increasing

the dose or switching the individual to another drug. Even though the drug is most often given for long periods of time, the effectiveness of long-term use has not been adequately studied.

CLINICAL TRIALS

The information on the effectiveness of Luvox in the manufacturer's clinical tests is presented here to demonstrate one major point. It's important to know that not all patients that take a drug will see an improvement in their symptoms. Just because the Food and Drug Administration (FDA) approves a drug and determines it to be safe and effective doesn't mean that it works in every patient who takes it. In fact, for many drugs, the number of patients that actually benefit from the drug and see a significant improvement in their disease or symptoms may be as low as 50 percent. This is not to say that the results presented should discourage patients from taking or trying Luvox, but that the same drug may produce different results in different patients. The solution to this dilemma is for the physician to keep trying several different medications until the most effective choice is found.

Major Depression

Researchers investigated the effectiveness of Luvox in several clinical studies, but the drug is not formally approved by the FDA for use in treating major depression. Luvox has been found to be significantly superior to a placebo (a placebo is defined as a pill with no medical properties) in improving the symptoms associated with major depressive illnesses. Patients in these studies saw an improvement in their depressed mood, as well as an improvement in the other symptoms associated with depression. There were, however, a small number of patients who did not see an improvement in their depression.

A comparison of the effectiveness of several different doses (50mg, 100mg, and 200mg) in treating depression have also been studied. These studies could not determine which particular dose was most effective in treating depression. Results varied from individual to individual. This means that the most effective dose for each patient must be individualized by a physician. Some patients may respond very well to a 50mg-per-day dose, while others may require a dose as high as 200mg. There is no magic dose in treating depression with Luvox.

Obsessive-Compulsive Disorder (OCD)

When Luvox was used to treat obsessive-compulsive disorder during two 10-week clinical studies, researchers found that patients' symptoms improved. Both studies found that Luvox was responsible for a significant improvement in the symptoms associated with OCD. Luvox was found to be just as effective in treating OCD regardless of age or gender. Other studies since that time have found similar results regarding effectiveness in treating OCD. The following table illustrates the results of study participants regarding their symptoms associated with OCD.

IMPROVEMENT IN SYMPTOMS ASSOCIATED WITH OCD

Outcome	No Drug	Luvox
Worse	6%	4%
No change	51%	31%
Minimally improved	32%	22%
Much improved	10%	30%
Very much improved	2%	13%

Slightly higher doses were used in the OCD clinical studies when compared to the depression clinical studies. This does not suggest, however, that higher doses should be used at the beginning of treatment with Luvox. Higher doses may be required, however, to effectively treat OCD as compared with depression. As always, the lowest possible dose that generates the most improvement in symptoms should always be the chosen dose for treatment of OCD.

CONTRAINDICATIONS

Luvox is extensively metabolized by the liver. This means that patients with liver diseases, even mild or stable cirrhosis or hepatitis, should be given a lower dose and/or take the drug less often. Patients with severe liver disease may want to be treated with a drug that is metabolized and excreted exclusively by the kidneys instead. Studies have been conducted with patients who have liver disease and who have been given Luvox. In patients with liver disease, the drug stayed in the body 30 percent longer and blood concentrations increased significantly. For patients with liver disease, doctors should choose initial doses and conduct any increases in dosage very cautiously. Therefore, individuals with liver problems or disorders should discuss this with their doctor before taking Luvox.

Patients with kidney disease should follow the same precautions as those with liver disease. Even though the drug is primarily metabolized by the liver, individuals with severe kidney problems may require smaller doses of Luvox, and they may need to take these doses less often. The effects of Luvox in patients with kidney disease or those who require renal dialysis have not been studied. Patients with kidney problems or disorders should discuss these issues with their doctor before taking Luvox.

Reports have cited serious and even fatal reactions in patients taking Luvox and MAO inhibitors such as Eldepryl, Furoxone, Matulane, Nardil, and Parnate. Some of these reactions have included high body temperature, rapid fluctuations of vital signs (high blood pressure and fast heartbeat), changes in mental status, extreme agitation, delirious behavior, and even coma. Some of these reactions have occurred as long as two weeks between the use of Luvox and Eldepryl, Furoxone, Matulane, Nardil, or Parnate. Therefore, patients should not begin Luvox therapy until at least two weeks after ceasing treatment with Eldepryl, Furoxone, Matulane, Nardil, or Parnate. If the patient has been using Luvox for long periods of time (greater than three months), he or she should not start treatment with these drugs until at least two to three weeks after treatment with Luvox has been stopped.

WARNINGS AND PRECAUTIONS

Luvox may cause adverse side effects that may be bothersome to some patients. The adverse effects that warrant special consideration usually occur in only a small number of individuals, but the seriousness of their consequences affords them special consideration and explanation. These side effects are not included in this book to frighten people taking Luvox, but more importantly to give them vital information based on the experiences of other patients.

During the clinical testing of Luvox, about 1 percent of the patients taking the drug experienced hypomania or mania. This adverse effect may aggravate or be bothersome to some individuals suffering from these conditions. Special consideration and monitoring should be given in patients who are diagnosed as bipolar or manic-depressive.

A small amount of weight loss and loss of appetite has occurred in patients taking Luvox. The weight loss associated with taking Luvox was less than five pounds. This effect, however, may be undesirable in some patients. Only very rarely have patients stopped taking Luvox because of weight loss or loss of appetite.

Patients who have experienced seizures or convulsions should also take precautions. The effect of Luvox on the frequency, duration, and severity of seizures and convulsions has not been extensively studied. No studies to date have examined the potential of the drug to increase the number of seizures in patients with epilepsy or other seizure disorders. However, in clinical trials for OCD, 0.2 percent (2 out of every 1,000 patients) experienced some sort of seizure. It is important to consider that other medications similar to Luvox have been known to cause seizures or convulsions in a small number of patients as well. Therefore, patients with epilepsy or a history of seizures or convulsions should be cautious when using Luvox.

A lot of media attention has focused on Prozac's purported ability to increase suicidal tendencies or drive patients to commit suicide. Patients may wonder if taking Luvox may cause the same suicidal tendencies because the two drugs are similar. Suicidal thoughts are one of the primary symptoms of depression, so it is hard to determine if it is the drug itself or the depressive episode that is the cause of suicidal thoughts and attempts. Until further studies can be conducted to determine the potential for Prozac or Luvox to cause suicidal thoughts, the conclusions about the increased risk of suicide while taking these drugs are questionable. The manufacturer of Prozac does, however, recommend close supervision of high-risk patients when beginning therapy with Prozac.

These same considerations should also be given to patients taking Luvox.

Clinical experience in patients with other chronic diseases who take Luvox is limited. Individuals with metabolic or blood disorders should also take precautions. There have been rare reports of blood disorders in patients taking Luvox. These reports include abnormal bleeding and purple spots on the skin, indicating broken blood vessels beneath the skin. Whether Luvox was solely responsible for these adverse effects was not clear.

Luvox has not been studied in patients with heart disease or who have suffered a heart attack. However, electrocardiograms (ECGs) in healthy individuals taking Luvox were normal (they did not show any significant abnormalities). There have been several cases of excessive sodium loss from the body or low sodium levels in patients taking Zoloft, Prozac, and Paxil. This condition is known as hyponatremia. Hyponatremia has not been specifically reported in patients taking Luvox. However, the risk of developing hyponatremia still exists. This condition, as with other electrolyte disturbances such as low potassium, may be serious especially in the elderly. The majority of these cases occurred in the elderly, with a few cases occurring in patients taking diuretics (water pills). The hyponatremia caused by Zoloft, Prozac, and Paxil is usually reversible once the drug is discontinued. Because Luvox is very similar to Zoloft, Prozac, and Paxil, these same precautions should be applied to its use as well.

USE IN THE ELDERLY

Luvox was found to be effective in treating depression in the elderly (patients sixty years and older) in several studies. However, elderly patients ages sixty-six to seventy-three exhibited a 40 percent higher concentration of the drug in the blood compared to younger patients (ages nineteen to thirty-five). Therefore, lower doses and smaller increases in those doses at longer intervals between increases may be necessary in elderly individuals. Also, older patients with serious medical conditions or those on multiple medications should discuss this with their doctor before taking Luvox. Multiple medical conditions may require smaller or less frequent doses of Luvox.

USE IN CHILDREN

Of the four drugs classified as SSRIs (Luvox, Prozac, Paxil, and Zoloft), Luvox is currently the only drug approved for use in treating children with OCD. The manufacturer examined the effectiveness in treating OCD in children in a ten-week study. Children between the ages of eight and seventeen were taking 50mg to 200mg per day depending on the severity of the disease in each child. Children in this study had moderate to severe OCD. The one shortcoming of the study was the relatively small number of children included. The following table illustrates the results of study participants regarding their symptoms associated with OCD.

IMPROVEMENT IN SYMPTOMS ASSOCIATED WITH OCD

Outcome	No Drug	Luvox
Worse	6%	8%
No change	44%	16%
Minimally improved	22%	37%
Much improved	17%	18%
Very much improved	11%	21%

The recommended dosage for children ages eight to seventeen is initially 25mg at bedtime. Doses of the drug may be increased in increments of 25mg per day every four to seven days. The normal range of doses in children is 50mg to 200mg per day. If the daily dose is more than 50mg, the dose should be equally divided in two. These higher doses should be taken in the morning and at bedtime. If the daily dose cannot be equally divided, the larger of the two doses should be taken at bedtime. The drug is not approved for use in children under the age of eight. For a more complete discussion on the use of Luvox and other SSRIs in children, refer to chapter 8, "Children and SSRIs."

AVERAGE RETAIL PRICES

The prices listed here are for informational purposes only. I present them to provide some basic information regarding the approximate cost of the drug Luvox. These prices are averages and may vary from pharmacy to pharmacy or within different regions of the country.

As is the case with some other prescription drugs, you might expect that the larger the dose, the larger the cost. Example: A 100mg tablet theoretically should cost twice as much as a 50mg tablet. For this particular class of drugs, the SSRIs, this is not the case. All three strengths of the drug cost the pharmacy approximately the same (within ten to twenty dollars per one hundred tablets) no matter what the strength. Therefore, prices for the 25mg, 50mg, and 100mg tablets may be somewhat similar.

Drug and Strength	Quantity	Retail Price
Luvox 25mg	30 tablets	$64.39–$78.49
Luvox 50mg	30 tablets	$67.69–$84.49
Luvox 100mg	30 tablets	$69.39–$85.98

SIDE EFFECTS

The side effects listed below were discovered during well-controlled clinical studies conducted before the FDA approved the drug for public use. Researchers believe the occurrence of these side effects under the drug's normal everyday use in real world settings to be very similar. Side effects are listed in decreasing order based on the percentage of patients experiencing certain side effects. The percentages listed below are averages based on several different clinic tests and are believed to be reliable.

Side Effect	Percentage Experiencing
Nausea/upset stomach	40%
Drowsiness	22%
Headache	22%
Insomnia	21%
Dry mouth	14%
Weakness	14%
Nervousness	12%
Dizziness	11%
Diarrhea	11%
Constipation	10%
Upper respiratory infection	9%
Abnormal ejaculation	8%
Increased sweating	7%
Loss of appetite	6%
Tremor	5%
Vomiting	5%
Gas	4%
Taste changes	3%
Increased urination	3%
Blurred vision	3%
Toothache, cavities, or abscess	3%
Flushed feeling	3%

Side Effect	Percentage Experiencing
Flulike symptoms	3%
Pounding heartbeat	3%
Impotence	2%
Difficulty swallowing	2%
Trouble breathing	2%
Increased yawning	2%
Decreased sex drive	2%
Depression	2%
Muscle tightness	2%
Agitation	2%
Chills	2%
Trouble having an orgasm	2%
Urinary retention	1%

The side effects listed above were reported by patients and, for the most part, were mild to moderate in severity. However, some side effects were severe enough for the patients taking Luvox to discontinue treatment. Some patients may have experienced more than one side effect. Overall, 22 percent of the patients taking Luvox in clinical trials stopped taking the drug due to side effects. The percentage of patients in clinical studies who stopped taking the drug as a result of a particular side effect are listed below.

Side Effect	Percentage Who Stopped Taking Luvox
Nausea	9%
Insomnia	4%
Drowsiness	4%
Headache	3%
Weakness	2%
Nervousness	2%
Dizziness	2%
Vomiting	2%

Side Effect	Percentage Who Stopped Taking Luvox
Stomach Pain	1%
Diarrhea	1%
Loss of appetite	1%
Dry mouth	1%

Researchers also discovered other side effects during clinical testing. These side effects occurred in a very small number of patients who had taken Luvox. Some of these side effects are very serious; it's important to remember, however, that only a very small number of patients taking Luvox even experienced these side effects. This should not discourage patients in any way from taking the drug Luvox. Many prescription drugs have most of these same side effects that occur infrequently or rarely with their use.

These side effects occurred in about 1 percent of the patients taking Luvox: accidental injury, tiredness, high blood pressure, low blood pressure, fast heartbeat, elevated liver enzymes, swelling, weight loss, weight gain, amnesia, absence of emotion, abnormal muscle movements, psychotic reaction, increased cough, and stuffy or runny nose.

The following list of side effects occurred infrequently (0.1 percent to 1 percent) in patients taking Luvox. (Note: 1 percent = 1 in every 100 patients and 0.1 percent = 1 in every 1,000 patients.)

allergic reaction
neck pain
neck stiffness
overdose
suicide attempt

increased skin sensitivity to
    sunburn
angina
slow heartbeat
cardiomyopathy

cold feet and hands
cardiovascular disease
pale skin
irregular heartbeat
colitis
increased belching
esophagitis
GI hemorrhage
swollen gums
hemorrhoids
rectal hemorrhage
decreased thyroid activity
anemia
swollen lymph nodes
low white blood cell count
dehydration
high cholesterol
muscle pain
arthritis
bursitis
muscle spasms
muscle numbness
convulsion
delusions
delirium
drug dependence
emotional instability
euphoria
hallucinations
hostility
hypochondria
hysteria
incoordination
increased saliva production

increased sex drive
nerve pain
sleep disorders
vertigo
twitching
psychosis
bloody nose
asthma
bronchitis
hoarseness
hyperventilation
itching
acne
discoloration of the skin
hair loss
eczema
scaly skin
dry skin
deafness
double vision
dry eyes
ear pain
eye pain
ear infection
loss of taste
breast pain
abnormal menstrual
   periods
abnormal breast milk
   production
menopause
urinary difficulties
vaginal hemorrhage
vaginitis

The following list of side effects occurred very rarely (0.1 percent to 0.001 percent or less) in patients taking Luvox. (Note: 0.1 percent = 1 in every 1,000 patients and 0.001 percent = 1 in every 100,000 patients.)

cyst

pelvic pain

sudden death

cerebrovascular accident

coronary artery disease

embolus

infection of the lining of the heart

loss of bloodflow to the lungs

gallbladder pain

trouble defecating

intestinal obstruction

jaundice

goiter

purple blotches on the skin

diabetes

high blood sugar

low blood sugar

low potassium

fractures

coma

obsessions

reflexes decreased

slurred speech

withdrawal syndrome

nasal congestion

hiccups

pneumonia

lung obstruction

eye ulcer

detached retina

decreased sperm production

These side effects are presented for information purposes only, not to scare individuals currently taking Luvox or to prevent them from taking it in the future. My hope is to increase the patient's awareness, and to report that in some rare instances the drug has caused serious side effects. Luvox and the SSRIs in general are some of the safest drugs on the market used to treat depression and OCD. However, you should discuss any abnormal side effects that you experience while taking Luvox with your physician and pharmacist.

DRUG INTERACTIONS

Compared with other drugs used to treat depression and OCD, Luvox and the SSRIs in general have fewer drug interactions. A drug interaction occurs when two drugs taken together produce an unwanted side effect or adverse effect, or when they affect how one drug or the other works in the body that is different from its intended use. The drug interactions listed below are the most clinically significant and potentially the most serious.

1. Luvox should never be taken with Eldepryl, Furoxone, Matulane, Nardil, or Parnate. This can cause a very serious and potentially life-threatening condition called serotonin syndrome. Symptoms of serotonin syndrome include mental status changes, confusion, restlessness, shivering, tremor, diarrhea, agitation, severe convulsions, and very high blood pressure. If serotonin syndrome is recognized early enough, the patient usually recovers quickly once these drugs are discontinued. There have been deaths, however, associated with this lethal combination. There is no actual treatment for serotonin syndrome, except for supportive care of body functions (maintaining adequate blood pressure, heart function, breathing, and so on).

    Patients taking Luvox should not take Eldepryl, Furoxone, Matulane, Nardil, or Parnate until at least two weeks after discontinuing treatment with Luvox. Conversely, patients who have taken Eldepryl, Furoxone, Matulane, Nardil, or Parnate should not be started on Luvox until at least two weeks after any of these drugs has been discontinued.

2. Luvox should not be taken with Propulsid or Hismanal. When Luvox and one of these drugs are taken together a serious and sometimes fatal irregular heartbeat may occur.

3. Luvox may increase the blood levels of Coumadin. Clinical studies showed that Luvox increased the blood levels of Coumadin by 98 percent. This may lead to increased bleeding, especially when Luvox is first started or recently discontinued, in patients taking Coumadin. This potential interaction can be very serious and may require your physician to adjust your dosage of Coumadin. Once the dosage of Coumadin is stabilized, Coumadin and Luvox can be taken safely together.

4. The amino acid tryptophan, contained in some vitamin supplements, should not be taken in large amounts with Luvox. Tryptophan is one of the chemicals that the body uses to make serotonin. SSRIs, like Luvox, increase the amount of serotonin available in the body. If a patient takes on excessive amount of tryptophan, the body may produce more serotonin than normal. This overproduction, along with Luvox's effect on serotonin, can result in excessive levels of serotonin. This may cause agitation, restlessness, insomnia, anxiety, and stomach problems like nausea, vomiting, and diarrhea. Therefore, vitamin supplements with large amounts of tryptophan should be avoided.

5. Luvox may increase the blood levels of Valium, Xanax, Halcion, and Versed. This may lead to decreased ability to think, memory problems, significant drowsiness, coordination problems, and many other unwanted side effects. These drugs should not be used together. It is, however, safe to take Luvox with other anti-anxiety medications such as Ativan, Serax, and Restoril.

6. Luvox may significantly increase the blood levels of theophylline-containing products such as Slo-Bid, Theo-Dur, Uniphyl, Uni-Dur, and others. If

Luvox and a theophylline-containing drug are used together, the dose of theophylline should be significantly reduced. The blood levels of theophylline should also be monitored very closely.

Other potential drug interactions are also worth mentioning. These interactions do not occur as frequently as the others listed above and are not nearly as serious.

1. Luvox may increase the drowsiness or sleepiness caused by alcohol, nerve medications, pain killers, muscle relaxers, antihistamines, allergy medications, cold medications, and cough syrups. This may be dangerous when driving, operating heavy machinery, or during any other task where mental alertness is required. This is not to say patients cannot take Luvox and these other drugs together. Patients just need to be aware that an increase in drowsiness may occur.

2. Luvox may increase the blood levels of Clozaril. The potential for Clozaril-related seizures and low blood pressure may be increased when taken with Luvox. Individuals taking Luvox and Clozaril together should monitor their blood glucose levels carefully.

3. Luvox may increase the blood levels of Tegretol. There have been some reports of toxic side effects when the two drugs are taken together. Individuals taking both Luvox and Tegretol together should be cautious of this potential interaction.

4. Luvox may alter the blood levels of lithium, which may lead to toxic effects. Blood levels of lithium should be measured and monitored. Seizures have been reported in patients taking lithium and Luvox together.

5. Luvox may increase the blood levels of other antidepressants such as Anafranil, Asendin, Elavil, Ludiomil, Norpramin, Pamelor, Sinequan, Sur-

montil, Tofranil, and Vivactil. This interaction
may increase the incidence of side effects associated with taking these antidepressants.

6. Luvox may increase the blood levels of Inderal
and Lopressor. There have been some reports of
toxic side effects, such as slow heart rate and low
blood pressure when the two drugs are taken together. Individuals taking both Luvox and either
Inderal or Lopressor should be cautious of this
potential interaction.

7. Luvox may increase the blood levels of methadone. There have been some reports of toxic side
effects, including extreme drowsiness, delirium,
and intoxication when the two drugs are taken
together. Individuals taking both Luvox and
methadone together should be cautious of this potential interaction.

8. Slow heart rate has been reported in patients taking Luvox and Cardizem, Cardizem SR, Cardizem CD, Dilacor XR, or Tiazac. This interaction
may be serious in some patients. Individuals taking Luvox and either of these medications should
be cautious of this potential interaction.

9. Luvox may increase the blood levels of caffeine
in the body. Caffeine causes nervousness and
stimulation and is found in coffee, tea, cola
drinks, and chocolate. Luvox is believed to cause
caffeine to stay in the body approximately eight
times longer than normal.

10. Recently, there have been rare reports of Luvox
causing weakness, muscle reflex problems, and
coordination problems when taken with Imitrex.
Individuals should be aware of this potential drug
interaction and use caution when taking Luvox
and Imitrex together.

Luvox was also tested with other drugs, including
Tenormin and Lanoxin, for potential drug interactions.

The tests found no drug interactions between these drugs and Luvox.

FOOD INTERACTIONS

Luvox may be taken with or without food or milk. Food or milk does not affect the amount of drug absorbed from the stomach and intestines. In fact, individuals who experience mild nausea from taking the drug on an empty stomach may wish to take it with food or milk.

DEALING WITH OVERDOSES

It is possible to overdose on Luvox when taking large quantities alone or with other drugs. The symptoms of an overdose include drowsiness, tiredness, nausea, vomiting, diarrhea, and dizziness. Two deaths have resulted when patients took Luvox alone in extremely large quantities. In the largest recorded overdose of Luvox at one time (10,000mg), the patient made a full recovery with no long-term effects from the overdose. Therefore, the risk of death from an overdose of Luvox alone should be considered extremely low. However, seventeen deaths have been associated with an overdose of Luvox when combined with other drug(s). If you suspect you or someone else have taken an overdose of Luvox, contact the nearest poison control center immediately.

ALLERGIES

Individuals who have a past history of being allergic to Luvox should not take the drug. Individuals allergic to other similar drugs in the same class, such as Prozac, Paxil, or Zoloft, should alert their doctor of this and use caution when taking Luvox. Most of the patients who experienced an allergic reaction reported only itching, hives, and a skin rash. However, some patients also reported fever, swollen glands, muscle pain, swelling, and/or trouble breathing. These symptoms disappeared in most patients once the drug was discontinued or when treated with antihistamines and/or steroids. If a rash, itching, swelling, fever, or swollen glands occurs while taking the drug, contact your doctor. If chest pain, difficulty in breathing, or the other symptoms listed above become worse, seek emergency medical treatment as quickly as possible.

CANCER-CAUSING POTENTIAL

There is no evidence that Luvox has the potential to cause cancer at this time, even at very high doses. Extensive testing in laboratory mice, hamsters, and rats found no evidence of cancer-causing potential in Luvox. These animals were given six times the normal human dose for periods of twenty to thirty months. Studies in these animals usually are good predictors of the likely effects in humans regarding cancer-causing potential.

EFFECT ON SEXUAL FUNCTION

Some evidence shows that Luvox has an effect on some sexual functions, including the ability to have an orgasm, the ability to maintain an erection, the ability to ejaculate, and sexual desire in general. In clinical testing, 8 percent of men taking the drug experienced some form of difficulty in ejaculating, 2 percent of men and women combined experienced a decrease in sexual desire, 2 percent of men noted impotence problems, and less than 1 percent of women experienced some other form of sexual dysfunction, possibly inability to have an orgasm. Individuals taking Luvox should be aware of these potential problems in sexual functioning and report them to their doctor if they become extremely bothersome.

EFFECT ON FERTILITY

There is no evidence that Luvox will cause fertility problems in either men or women. Fertility studies in both male and female rats taking two times the maximum human dose showed no effect on mating performance, duration of gestation, or pregnancy rate. It is important to realize that there are risks associated with taking any drug if a woman believes she is pregnant. If a woman suspects she is pregnant, she should obtain a pregnancy test immediately and discuss with her physician whether she should continue taking Luvox or not. For a complete discussion on the effects of the drug during pregnancy, see the following section.

SAFETY OF USE DURING PREGNANCY

Luvox is classified under the Food and Drug Administration's Pregnancy Classification as Category C. Category C means animal studies have shown an adverse effect on an animal fetus. However, no one has conducted adequate studies in humans, but the benefits of taking the drug during pregnancy must truly outweigh the risks based on the results of animal testing. Some animal studies using as much as two times the maximum daily dose of Luvox showed some harm to the unborn fetus. However, other animal studies on rats showed an increase in the number of stillborn young, a decrease in total birth weight, and an increase in the number of young surviving after birth. It is important to know that extensive studies on the effect of Luvox on the human fetus have not been done. If you suspect that you are pregnant, contact your doctor immediately. The manufacturer strongly recommends that Luvox be used during pregnancy only if the benefits of taking the drug significantly outweigh the risks of potential harm to the fetus.

SAFETY OF USE WHEN BREAST-FEEDING

Luvox is excreted in the breast milk. The concentration of the drug in breast milk is similar to that found in the mother's bloodstream. We lack well-controlled studies regarding the effect on the infant of breast milk containing Luvox. Therefore, in the best interest of the infant, mothers should never breast-feed while taking the drug.

EXCRETION FROM THE BODY

Luvox is extensively metabolized by the liver and is removed from the body by the kidneys. This process is slow, which results in the drug staying in the body for quite some time. In fact, the drug will stay in the body for about sixteen hours after taking a single dose and one to two days after several days of therapy with Luvox. Luvox is metabolized by the liver into various inactive chemical compounds. These chemical compounds are not considered active in treating depression and OCD. Patients who have been taking the drug for several weeks should not expect the body to be free of the drug until about one week after taking the last dose.

WHAT TO KNOW BEFORE YOU USE THIS DRUG

Because the drug is metabolized by the liver, patients with liver disease, hepatitis, or cirrhosis may require lower doses. Physicians should make the same consideration for patients with kidney disease. Lower doses may be required in these patients as well. Also, patients who suffer from seizure disorders or epilepsy may want to inform their doctor of this condition before taking Luvox. The weight loss that occurs rarely when taking Luvox should be considered carefully. In some patients, this side effect may be undesirable.

Luvox is not considered a "quick fix" in treating depression or OCD. The drug may require several weeks of therapy before a significant improvement is seen. Therefore, patients should not become discouraged if immediate improvements are not seen and quit taking the drug. The drug should be taken for at least four to six weeks before the patient and his or her physician decide the drug is not working and that some other medication should be used.

PROPER USE OF THE DRUG

Luvox should be taken every day in order to receive its maximum benefits. The patient should follow the dosing schedule set by his or her physician as closely as possible. Do not take more or less of the drug than is prescribed. Some patients may try to increase the dose on their own if they feel the drug is not effective at the prescribed dose. This may increase the risk of unwanted side effects and other adverse events. Other patients may try to decrease their dose on their own if they experience some unwanted side effects. This may result in too low of a dose being taken. Patients experiencing any unwanted side effects or who feel that the current dose may be too low should discuss this with their physician or pharmacist before adjusting the amount of medication taken.

If a patient forgets to take his or her daily dose and remembers within two to four hours of when the dose was to be taken, the patient should take the drug as soon as he or she remembers. If the patient forgets to take his or her daily dose and remembers more than four hours after the medication time, he or she should skip the missed dose and continue on the normal dosing schedule the next day or take the next scheduled dose on time. Patients should not double the dose.

IMPORTANT PATIENT INFORMATION

Individuals taking Luvox should make regular visits to their physician to check and discuss the progress of their condition. At that time, patients should report any side effects or other adverse effects to their physician. If a skin rash, itching, or hives occur after taking the drug, stop taking the drug and contact your physician as soon as possible. These may be the signs and symptoms of an allergic reaction to the drug. If these symptoms are accompanied by tightness in the chest or trouble breathing, seek medical attention immediately.

Luvox may cause some drowsiness and tiredness, especially at first. The degree of drowsiness caused by Luvox is significantly less severe than that caused by pain killers, sleeping pills, and other nerve medications. Patients should use caution when driving, operating heavy machinery or equipment, or doing jobs that require a great deal of mental alertness. Therefore, when taking the drug for the first few doses, patients should be cautious of its potential to cause drowsiness and observe how it affects them personally. The degree of drowsiness caused by the drug varies from patient to patient.

It is also important to know that alcohol, nerve medications, pain killers, muscle relaxers, antihistamines, allergy and cold medications, cough syrups, and other drugs known to cause drowsiness may significantly increase the drowsiness caused by Luvox. Therefore extreme caution should be used when Luvox is taken with these drugs. The drug may also cause some limited dizziness or lightheadedness, especially when getting up suddenly from lying or sitting positions.

Some patients taking Luvox may experience a dry mouth for a short period of time. This side effect is similar in severity to the dry mouth caused by some antihistamines. This side effect can be alleviated by chewing sugarless gum or candy. If the dry mouth continues for more than two weeks, patients should contact their physician.

If stomach upset or mild nausea occurs after taking Luvox, the patient may take it with food or milk to reduce this irritating side effect. If the nausea or stomach upset is severe, continues every time the drug is taken for several days, or vomiting occurs, contact your physician or pharmacist.

Many times Luvox is prescribed to be taken at bedtime. Food and milk do not significantly affect the action of the drug in the body or its absorption in the stomach. Therefore, the drug may be taken with a late evening snack or on an empty stomach.

STORAGE OF THE DRUG

Luvox, like all medications, should be kept out of the reach of children. Store the drug away from direct light and heat. Never store any medication in a bathroom medicine cabinet. Heat, moisture, and steam from the shower, bathtub, and sink may cause medications to become ineffective. Medications should also not be stored near the kitchen sink or in any other damp place for the same reason. Ideally, your prescription medications should be stored in a tight, light-resistant (amber or brown) prescription bottle between 59 and 86 degrees and at no more than 104 degrees. Medications are best stored in the original bottles in which they were dispensed. Remember, the temperatures in a hot car or truck can exceed 105 degrees very easily. Therefore, medications should never be left in a hot car or truck for more than thirty to sixty minutes.

FURTHER INFORMATION

Individuals who would like further information on Luvox should first contact their pharmacist and then their physician. Another source of in-depth information is your local hospital. Many large hospitals, especially those associated with universities, have drug information centers. When calling the hospital, ask for the pharmacy department or drug information center of the hospital. Finally, individuals can contact the company that manufactures and markets the drug directly. Solvay Pharmaceuticals Inc., which manufactures Luvox, can be reached at this address: Solvay Pharmaceuticals, ATT: Medical Services Department, 901 Sawyer Road, Marietta, GA 30062. The phone number is (770) 578-9000 or (800) 354-0026.

FOUR

❧

Paxil

BRAND NAME

The brand name of the drug is Paxil.

GENERIC NAME

The generic name of the drug is paroxetine. Currently no generic form is available. The patent on the drug should expire sometime after the year 2000. By this time, a generic alternative will probably become available.

DOSAGE FORMS

Paxil is available in 10mg, 20mg, 30mg, and 40mg tablets. The drug is currently not available in a liquid form.

APPROVED AND ACCEPTED USES

Paxil has been approved for use in adult patients with major depression. A major depression episode is defined as a persistent depressed mood that interferes with daily functioning nearly every day for at least two weeks. It should also include at least four of the following eight symptoms: change in appetite, change in sleep, loss of interest in usual activities, decreased sex drive, increased feeling of tiredness, feeling of guilt or worthlessness, slowed thinking or impaired concentration, and a suicide attempt or thoughts of suicide.

Paxil has also been approved for use in obsessive-compulsive disorder (OCD). OCD is defined as obsessions or compulsions that cause extreme distress, are time-consuming, or significantly interfere with functioning socially or at work. The patient recognizes these behaviors as excessive and unreasonable, but still cannot control the urge to perform them.

Paxil has also been approved for use in panic disorder. This may or may not include symptoms of agoraphobia (the fear of being in open or public places). Panic disorder is characterized by the occurrence of unexpected and recurrent panic attacks. Panic attacks usually have a discrete period of intense fear or discomfort that develops abruptly and reach a peak within ten minutes. During this time, there is a sudden feeling of intense apprehension, fearfulness, terror, and/or impending doom. Panic attacks also usually include at least four or more of the following symptoms:

1. pounding heartbeat or increased heart rate
2. intense sweating
3. trembling or shaking
4. sensations of shortness of breath or feeling smothered
5. feeling of choking
6. chest pain or discomfort
7. nausea or stomach distress
8. feeling dizzy, unsteady, lightheaded, or faint
9. feelings of unreality or being detached from oneself
10. fear of losing control

11. fear of dying
12. numbness or tingling sensations
13. chills or hot flashes

These attacks may also include the associated concern about having additional attacks, worrying about the implications or consequences of the attacks, and/or a significant change in behavior related to the attacks.

USUAL DOSE

The usual dose in treating depression is 20mg to 50mg daily. Usually patients take Paxil in the morning as a single dose. Studies have been conducted to test the effectiveness of 10mg to 50mg daily doses. Most patients are started on a 20mg-per-day dose. In patients with severe cases, doses as high as 50mg per day may be needed in order to obtain the desired antidepressive effect. Doses of Paxil may be increased to a maximum of 50mg per day by a physician after several weeks if the patient sees no significant improvement of the symptoms. Physicians should wait at least one week between dosage increases. Individuals should not take more than 50mg of Paxil per day. The drug may require several weeks of treatment before patients see noticeable improvement. Therefore, individuals should not expect immediate results or a spontaneous miracle when taking the drug. Limited research studies have shown that Paxil is effective in treating depression for time periods as long as one year. Other evidence suggests that Paxil is effective in treating depression for longer periods of time.

The usual dose in treating obsessive-compulsive disorder (OCD) is 40mg once daily in the morning. Patients are usually started on 20mg daily with dosage increases of 10mg per day at one-week intervals until the desired effect is seen. The doctor may prescribe higher doses of up to 60mg per day if, after several weeks of treatment with lower doses, the patient sees no improvement. The maximum dose of Paxil for treating OCD is 60mg daily.

The usual dose in treating panic disorder is 40mg once daily in the morning. Patients should be started on 10mg once daily and increased 10mg per week until the desired effect is seen. The doctor may prescribe higher doses of up to 60mg per day if, after several weeks of treatment with lower doses, the patient sees no improvement. The maximum dose of Paxil for treating panic disorder is 60mg.

ONSET OF ACTIVITY AND LENGTH OF ACTION

After a patient takes a single dose of Paxil, the drug stays in the body for approximately twenty-one hours. After several days of use, the drug stays in the body approximately forty-two hours. It usually takes between one to four weeks before patients see noticeable improvement in symptoms. In some individuals the time period for improvement may be several weeks or even a few months. Patients usually see improvement in sleep patterns in as little as one to two weeks. If the patient sees no improvement after several weeks, the physician may want to consider increasing the dose or switching the individual to another drug. Even though the drug is most often given for long periods of time, the effectiveness of long-term use has not been adequately studied.

CLINICAL TRIALS

The information on the effectiveness of Paxil in the manufacturer's clinical tests is presented here to demonstrate one major point. It's important to know that not all patients who take a drug will see an improvement in their symptoms. Just because the Food and Drug Administration (FDA) has approved a drug and determined it to be safe and effective doesn't mean that it works in every patient who takes it. In fact, for many drugs, the number of patients that actually benefit from the drug and see a significant improvement in their disease or symptoms may be as low as 50 percent. This is not to say that the results presented should discourage patients from taking or trying Paxil, but that the same drug may produce different results in different patients. The solution to this dilemma is for the physician to keep trying several different medications until the most effective choice is found.

MAJOR DEPRESSION

The manufacturer investigated the effectiveness of Paxil in several clinical studies before the FDA approved the drug for public use. Other similar clinical studies, conducted since FDA approval, have demonstrated many of the same results in treating depression. Paxil was shown to be significantly superior to a placebo (a placebo is a pill with no medical properties) in improving the symptoms associated with major depressive illnesses in patients ages eighteen to seventy-three. Patients in these studies saw an improvement in their depressed mood as well as an improvement in sleep disturbances and anxiety. A small number of patients, however, did not see an improvement in their depression.

A large number of patients from the short-term-use studies of Paxil were included in another study to determine the drug's effectiveness over longer periods of time. One group of patients continued taking the drug for a period of one year while another group took a placebo. In the group that continued taking Paxil, only 15 percent had a major depressive relapse compared to 39 percent of the placebo group during that one-year time period.

OBSESSIVE-COMPULSIVE DISORDER

When Paxil was tested to treat obsessive-compulsive disorder (OCD), two 12-week clinical studies found that symptoms did improve. Patients in these studies were diagnosed with moderate to severe OCD. Both studies found that Paxil was responsible for a significant improvement in the symptoms associated with OCD. The first study tested doses of 20mg, 40mg, and 60mg per day. Only the 40mg and 60mg doses were found to be effective in treating OCD. This study was also extended to determine the effectiveness in treating OCD over the long term. Patients taking the drug for as long as one year saw significant improvement. The second study, which combined the use of Paxil with Anafranil, found similar results. Also, researchers saw no differences in effectiveness based on age or gender of the patient. Other studies since that time have found similar results regarding effectiveness in treating OCD. The following table illustrates the results of study participants regarding their symptoms associated with OCD.

IMPROVEMENT IN SYMPTOMS ASSOCIATED WITH OCD

Outcome	No Drug	20mg Paxil	40mg Paxil	60mg Paxil
Worse	14%	7%	7%	3%
No change	44%	35%	22%	19%
Minimally improved	24%	33%	29%	34%
Much improved	11%	18%	22%	24%
Very much improved	7%	7%	20%	20%

Slightly higher doses were used in the OCD clinical studies when compared to the depression clinical studies. This does not suggest, however, that higher doses should be used at the beginning of treatment with Paxil. But higher doses may be required to effectively treat OCD as compared with depression. However, physicians should always choose the lowest possible dose where the most improvement in symptoms is seen for treatment of OCD.

Panic Disorder

Three separate clinical tests studied the drug's effectiveness in treating panic disorder. In the first study, 76 percent of the patients taking 40mg of Paxil daily were free of panic attacks compared to only 44 percent in the placebo group. Patients taking 10mg or 20mg of Paxil did not see a significant improvement in the number of panic attacks or their symptoms. In the second study, 51 percent of the patients taking Paxil were free of panic attacks compared to only 32 percent in the placebo group. In the third study, 33 percent of the patients taking Paxil experienced either zero or one panic attacks compared to only 14 percent in the placebo group. The patients in this study were also receiving behavioral therapy as well. In studies two and three, patients were taking a variety of different doses (10mg to 60mg) of Paxil, but the average dose was 40mg per day. Longer-term studies of up to one year in length did show a significant reduction in the number and severity of panic attacks as well.

CONTRAINDICATIONS

Paxil is metabolized by the liver. This means that patients with liver diseases, even mild or stable cirrhosis or hepatitis, should take a lower dose and/or take the drug less often. Patients with severe liver disease may want to be treated with a drug that is metabolized and excreted exclusively by the kidneys instead. Studies have been conducted with patients who have liver disease and who have been given Paxil. In patients with liver disease, the drug stayed in the body longer and blood concentrations doubled compared to those with normal liver function. Therefore, individuals with liver problems or disorders should discuss this with their doctor before taking Paxil.

Patients with kidney disease should follow the same precautions as those with liver disease. Even though the drug is primarily metabolized by the liver, the drug is primarily excreted by the kidneys in the urine. In individuals with poor kidney function, the drug concentration in the blood may increase fourfold. Therefore, individuals with severe kidney problems may require smaller doses of Paxil and those doses may need to be given less often. The effects of Paxil in patients with kidney disease or those who require renal dialysis has not been studied. Therefore, individuals with kidney problems or disorders should discuss these issues with their doctor before taking Paxil.

There have been reports of serious and even fatal reactions in patients taking Paxil and MAO inhibitors such as Eldepryl, Furoxone, Matulane, Nardil, and Parnate. Some of these reactions have included high body temperature, rapid fluctuations of vital signs (high blood pressure and fast heartbeat), changes in mental status, extreme agitation, delirious behavior, and even coma. Some of these reactions have occurred as long as two weeks between the use of Paxil and Eldepryl, Furoxone, Matulane, Nardil, or Parnate. Therefore, patients should not start Paxil therapy until at least two weeks after they have stopped taking Eldepryl, Furoxone, Matulane, Nardil, or Parnate. If the patient has been using Paxil for long periods of time (longer than three months), he or she should not start treatment with these drugs until at least two to three weeks after treatment with Paxil has been stopped.

WARNINGS AND PRECAUTIONS

Paxil may cause adverse effects that may be bothersome to some patients. The adverse effects that warrant special consideration usually occur in only a small number of individuals, but the seriousness of their consequences affords them special consideration and explanation. These side effects are not included in this book to frighten people currently taking Paxil, but more importantly to give them vital information based on the experiences of other patients.

In some clinical testing of Paxil for depression, 1 percent of the patients experienced hypomania or mania. In patients who are classified as bipolar, 2 percent experienced a manic episode. This adverse effect may aggravate or be bothersome to some individuals suffering from these conditions. Special consideration and monitoring should be given in patients who are diagnosed as bipolar or manic-depressive.

A small amount of weight loss and loss of appetite has occurred in patients taking Paxil. The weight loss associated with taking Paxil was about 1 pound. This effect, however, may be undesirable in some patients. Only very rarely have patients stopped taking Paxil because of weight loss or loss of appetite.

Patients who have experienced seizures or convulsions should also take precautions. In clinical studies, seizures occurred in only 0.1 percent (1 patient in every 1,000). This rate is similar to that of other drugs used to treat depression. Nevertheless, patients with epilepsy or a history of seizures or convulsions should be cautious when using Paxil.

A lot of media attention has focused on Prozac's purported ability to increase suicidal tendencies or drive patients to commit suicide. Patients may wonder if taking Paxil may cause the same suicidal tendencies because the two drugs are similar. Suicidal thoughts are one of the primary symptoms of depression, so it is hard to determine if it is the drug itself or the depressive episode that is the cause for suicidal thoughts and attempts. Until further studies can be conducted to determine the potential for Prozac or Paxil to cause suicidal thoughts, the conclusions about the increased risk of suicide while taking these drugs are questionable. The manufacturer of Paxil does, however, recommend close supervision of high-risk patients when beginning therapy with Paxil.

Clinical experience in patients with other chronic diseases who have taken Paxil is limited. Paxil has not been studied in patients with heart disease or in those who have suffered a heart attack. However, electrocardiograms (ECGs) in healthy individuals taking Paxil were normal (they did not show any significant abnormalities). Other vital signs such as blood pressure, pulse, body temperature, and liver function tests were also all normal in healthy individuals who took Paxil. However, Paxil should be used very cautiously in patients with metabolic or blood disorders.

Paxil has been associated with abnormal bleeding in several reports. Most of these cases have been minor in nature, but there have been reports of altered platelet function. These reports include patients experiencing abnormal bleeding and purple spots on the skin, indicating broken blood vessels beneath the skin. Whether or not Paxil is solely responsible for these adverse effects has not been determined.

Several cases of excessive sodium loss from the body or low sodium levels have occurred in patients taking Paxil. This condition is known as hyponatremia. This condition, like other electrolyte disturbances such as low potassium, may be serious, especially in the elderly. The majority of these cases occurred in the elderly, and some patients were taking diuretics (water pills). The hyponatremia caused by Paxil is usually reversible once the drug is discontinued.

USE IN THE ELDERLY

The use of Paxil in elderly patients (sixty years and older) with depression has been studied. The drug was found to be effective in treating depression in this group of patients. However, concentrations of Paxil in the blood were 70 percent to 80 percent higher in elderly patients when compared to nonelderly patients. Therefore, initial doses in the elderly should be lower and dosage increases carefully monitored. Also, older patients with serious medical conditions or those on multiple medications should discuss this with their doctor. These conditions may also require smaller or less frequent doses of Paxil.

USE IN CHILDREN

Paxil is currently not approved for use in children. This does not mean, however, that physicians are not prescribing the drug for children. The manufacturer has not conducted any well-controlled studies regarding Paxil's use in children. For a complete discussion on the use of Paxil and other SSRIs in children, refer to Chapter 8, "Children and SSRIs."

AVERAGE RETAIL PRICES

The prices listed here are for informational purposes only. I present them to provide some basic information regarding the approximate cost of the drug Paxil. These prices are averages and may vary from pharmacy to pharmacy or within different regions of the country.

As is the case with some other prescription drugs, you might expect that the larger the dose, the larger the cost. Example: A 20mg tablet theoretically should cost twice as much as a 10mg tablet. For this particular class of drugs, the SSRIs, this is not the case. All three strengths of the drug cost the pharmacy approximately the same (within ten to twenty dollars per one hundred tablets) no matter what the strength. Therefore, prices for the 10mg, 20mg, 30mg, and 40mg tablets may be somewhat similar.

Drug and Strength	Quantity	Retail Price
Paxil 10mg	30 tablets	$59.85–$81.50
Paxil 20mg	30 tablets	$60.69–$86.51
Paxil 30mg	30 tablets	$63.39–$87.98
Paxil 40mg	30 tablets	$66.69–$90.51

SIDE EFFECTS

The side effects listed below were discovered during well-controlled clinical studies conducted before the FDA approved the drug for public use. Researchers believe the occurrence of these side effects under the drug's normal everyday use in real world settings to be very similar. Side effects are listed in decreasing order based on the percentage of patients experiencing certain side effects. The percentages listed below are averages based on several different clinical tests and are believed to be reliable.

Side Effect	Percentage Experiencing
Nausea/upset stomach	23%–26%
Drowsiness	23%–24%
Headache	18%
Dry mouth	18%
Weakness	15%–22%
Constipation	14%–16%
Trouble ejaculating	13%–23%
Insomnia	13%–24%
Dizziness	12%–13%
Diarrhea	10%–12%
Sexual dysfunction in males	10%
Increased sweating	9%–11%
Tremors	8%–11%
Impotence in males	8%
Decreased appetite	6%–9%
Nervousness	5%–9%
Increased appetite	4%
Numbness	4%
Gas	4%
Increased yawning	4%
Abnormal vision	4%
Blurred vision	4%
Abnormal dreams	4%
Decreased sex drive	3%–7%
Increased urination	3%
Trouble concentrating	3%
Difficulty urinating	3%
Sexual dysfunction in females	2%–3%
Pounding heartbeat	2%–3%
Rash	2%–3%
Taste changes	2%
Drugged feeling	2%
Feeling of a lump in the throat	2%
Extreme muscle tension	2%

Side Effect	Percentage Experiencing
Amnesia	2%
Confusion	1%
Muscle pain	1%
Muscle numbness	1%

The side effects listed above were reported by patients and, for the most part, were mild to moderate in severity. However, some side effects were severe enough for the patients taking Paxil to discontinue treatment. In fact, about 10 percent of the patients taking Paxil during clinical testing did stop taking the drug due to side effects. Those side effects that caused patients to stop taking the drug were drowsiness, insomnia, nervousness, tremors, dizziness, nausea, constipation, diarrhea, dry mouth, vomiting, muscle weakness, increased sweating, impotence, and ejaculation problems. Some patients who discontinued taking Paxil due to side effects experienced more than one of those listed above.

Researchers also discovered other side effects during clinical testing. These side effects occurred in a very small number of patients who had taken Paxil. Some of these side effects are very serious; it's important to remember, however, that only a very small number of patients taking Paxil even experienced these side effects. This should not discourage patients in any way from taking the drug Paxil. Many prescription drugs have most of these same side effects that occur infrequently or rarely with their use.

These side effects occurred in about 1 percent of the patients taking Paxil: chills, weight gain, weight loss, tiredness, ringing in the ears, increased cough, runny nose, and itching.

The following list of side effects occurred infrequently (0.1 percent to 1 percent) in patients taking Paxil. (Note:

1 percent = 1 in every 100 patients and 0.1 percent = 1 in every 1,000 patients.)

allergic reaction
face swelling
cancer
neck pain
slow heartbeat
irregular heartbeat
low blood pressure
migraines
colitis
teeth grinding
increased belching
increased salivation
swollen gums
abnormal liver function tests
mouth sores
stomach ulcers
anemia
low white blood cell count
purple spots on the skin
high blood sugar
swelling in the legs
increased thirst
high levels of potassium in
  the blood
high cholesterol
gout
low blood sugar
high levels of calcium in the
  blood

abnormal thinking
movement difficulties
convulsions
hallucinations
lack of coordination
lack of emotion
limited paralysis
paranoid reaction
asthma
bronchitis
difficulty breathing
bloody nose
hyperventilation
flu
stuffy nose
changes in voice
ear pain
eye pain
ear infection
loss of taste
acne
dry skin
hair loss
eczema
abortion
breast pain
abnormal menstrual periods
vaginal infections
urinary difficulties

The following list of side effects occurred very rarely (0.001 percent to 0.1 percent or less) in patients taking Paxil. (Note: 0.1percent = 1 in every 1,000 patients and

0.001 percent = 1 in every 100,000 patients taking Paxil.)

abscess
pelvic pain
ulcers
neck stiffness
bloody diarrhea
bulimia
bowel impaction
bleeding gums
hepatitis
tongue discoloration
swollen tongue
tooth abnormalities
cavities
diabetes
changes in thyroid function
angina
congestive heart failure
heart attack
pale skin
varicose veins
bursitis
osteoporosis
muscle spasms

muscle cramps
delirium
delusions
double vision
convulsions
increased sex drive
manic-depressive reaction
decreased reflexes
withdrawal syndrome
skin discoloration
increased sensitivity of the
   skin to sunlight
enlarged breasts in both
   males and females
breast cancer
breast milk production
skin ulcers
dry skin
dandruff
cataracts
deafness
kidney pain

These side effects are presented for information purposes only, not to scare individuals currently taking Paxil or to prevent them from taking it in the future. My hope is to increase the patient's awareness, and to report that in some rare instances the drug has caused serious side effects. Paxil and the SSRIs in general are some of the safest drugs on the market used to treat depression and OCD. However, you should discuss any abnormal side effects that you experience while taking Paxil with your physician and pharmacist.

DRUG INTERACTIONS

Compared with other drugs used to treat depression and OCD, Paxil and the SSRIs in general have fewer drug interactions. A drug interaction occurs when two drugs taken together produce an unwanted side effect or adverse effect, or when they affect how one drug or the other works in the body that is different from its intended use. The drug interactions listed below are the most clinically significant and potentially the most serious.

1. Paxil should never be taken with Eldepryl, Furoxone, Matulane, Nardil, or Parnate. This can cause a very serious and potentially life-threatening condition called serotonin syndrome. Symptoms of serotonin syndrome include mental status changes, confusion, restlessness, shivering, tremor, diarrhea, agitation, severe convulsions, and very high blood pressure. If serotonin syndrome is recognized early enough, the patient usually recovers quickly once these drugs are discontinued. However, there have been deaths associated with this lethal combination. Physicians administer no actual treatment for serotonin syndrome, except for supportive care of body functions (maintaining adequate blood pressure, heart function, breathing, etc.).

   Patients taking Paxil should not take Eldepryl, Furoxone, Matulane, Nardil, or Parnate until at least two weeks after discontinuing treatment with Paxil. Conversely, patients who have taken Eldepryl, Furoxone, Matulane, Nardil, or Parnate should not be started on Paxil until at least two weeks after any of these drugs has been discontinued.

2. Paxil may increase the blood levels of the drug Coumadin. This may lead to increased bleeding, especially when Paxil is first started or recently discontinued, in patients taking Coumadin. This potential interaction can be very serious and may require your physician to adjust your dosage of Coumadin. Once the dosage of Coumadin is stabilized, Coumadin and Paxil can be taken safely together.

3. The amino acid tryptophan, contained in some vitamin supplements, should not be taken in large amounts with Paxil. Tryptophan is one of the chemicals that serotonin is made from in the body. SSRIs like Paxil increase the amount of serotonin available in the body. If a patient takes an excessive amount of tryptophan, the body may produce more serotonin than normal. This overproduction, along with Paxil's effect on serotonin, can result in excessive levels of serotonin. This may cause agitation, restlessness, insomnia, anxiety, and stomach problems like nausea, vomiting, and diarrhea. Therefore, vitamin supplements with large amounts of tryptophan should be avoided.

Other potential drug interactions are also worth mentioning. These interactions do not occur as frequently as those listed above and are not nearly as serious.

1. Paxil may increase the drowsiness or sleepiness caused by alcohol, nerve medications, pain killers, muscle relaxers, antihistamines, allergy medications, cold medications, and cough syrups. This may be dangerous when driving, operating heavy machinery, or during any other task requiring mental alertness. This is not to say patients cannot take Paxil and these other drugs together. Patients just need to be aware that an increase in drowsiness may occur.

2. Phenobarbital may decrease the blood levels of Paxil. This may require only a slight adjustment in the patient's dosage of Paxil or may not require any dosage adjustment at all. The patient's physician will assess the clinical effectiveness of a dosage adjustment.

3. Tagamet may increase the blood levels of Paxil. Individuals taking Tagamet and Paxil together should be cautious of this potential interaction.

4. Dilantin may decrease the blood levels of Paxil, possibly leading to low blood sugar in some individuals. This may require only a slight adjustment in the patient's dosage of Paxil taken or may not require any dosage adjustment at all. The patient's physician will assess the clinical effectiveness of a dosage adjustment.

5. Paxil may alter the blood levels of lithium, which may lead to toxic effects. Blood levels of lithium should be measured and monitored.

6. Paxil may increase the blood levels of other antidepressants such as Anafranil, Asendin, Elavil, Ludiomil, Norpramin, Pamelor, Sinequan, Surmontil, Tofranil, and Vivactil. This interaction may increase the incidence of side effects associated with taking these antidepressants.

7. Recently, there have been rare reports of Paxil causing weakness, muscle reflex problems, and coordination problems when taken with Imitrex. Individuals should be aware of this potential drug interaction and use caution when taking Paxil and Imitrex together.

8. Paxil may increase the blood levels of Kemadrin. This may require the dose of Kemadrin to be reduced.

9. Paxil has been shown to increase the blood levels of theophylline drugs such as Slo-Bid, Theo-Dur,

Uniphyl, Uni-Dur, and others. Physicians should monitor theophylline blood levels in patients taking Paxil.

Paxil was also tested with Inderal and Valium for potential drug interactions. Although these tests found no interactions with these drugs, Valium may increase the drowsiness caused by Paxil.

FOOD INTERACTIONS

Paxil may be taken with or without food or milk. Food, milk, or antacids do not affect the amount of drug absorbed from the stomach and intestines. In fact, individuals who experience mild nausea from taking the drug on an empty stomach may wish to take it with food or milk.

DEALING WITH OVERDOSES

It is possible to overdose on Paxil when taking large quantities alone or with other drugs and/or alcohol. The symptoms of an overdose include nausea, vomiting, sedation, dizziness, sweating, and facial flushness. There have been no reports of coma or convulsions when Paxil was taken alone in an overdose. However, deaths have been reported (rarely) when patients took Paxil with other drugs or alone in very large doses. Therefore, the risk of death from an overdose of Paxil alone should be considered low. If you suspect that you or someone else have taken an overdose of Paxil, contact your nearest poison control center immediately.

ALLERGIES

Individuals who have a past history of being allergic to Paxil should not take the drug. Individuals allergic to other similar drugs in the same class, such as Prozac,

Zoloft, or Luvox, should alert their doctor of this and use caution when taking Paxil. Most of the patients who experienced an allergic reaction reported only itching and a skin rash. However, some patients also reported fever, swollen glands, muscle pain, swelling, and/or trouble breathing. These symptoms disappeared in most patients once the drug was discontinued or when treated with antihistamines and/or steroids. If a rash, itching, swelling, fever, or swollen glands occurs while taking the drug, contact your doctor. If chest pain, difficulty in breathing, or the other symptoms listed above become worse, seek emergency medical treatment as quickly as possible.

CANCER-CAUSING POTENTIAL

There is no evidence that Paxil has the potential to cause cancer at this time, even at very high doses. Extensive testing in laboratory mice found no evidence of cancer-causing potential in Paxil. Studies in mice usually are good predictors of the likely effects in humans regarding cancer-causing potential.

EFFECT ON SEXUAL FUNCTION

Some evidence shows that Paxil has an effect on some sexual functions, including the ability to have an orgasm, the ability to maintain an erection, the ability to ejaculate, and sexual desire in general. In clinical testing, 13 percent to 23 percent of men taking the drug experienced some form of difficulty in ejaculating, 3 percent to 7 percent of the men and women combined experienced a decrease in sexual desire, 8 percent of men noted impotence problems, and 2 percent to 3 percent of the women experienced some other form of sexual dysfunction, possibly inability to have an orgasm. Two percent of the men taking the drug during clinical testing felt the problem of difficulty in ejaculating during sex was severe enough for them to stop taking the drug. Individuals taking Paxil should be aware of these potential problems in sexual functioning and report them to their doctor if they become extremely bothersome.

EFFECT ON FERTILITY

There is no direct evidence that Paxil will cause fertility problems in either men or women. However, studies did show a decrease in fertility in both male and female rats. Rats in these studies received a dose of Paxil fifteen times greater than a human dose. Female rats saw a decrease in pregnancy rates, and male rats exhibited irreversible lesions in the male reproduction organs, which caused infertility. Risks are associated with taking any drug if a woman believes she is pregnant. If a woman suspects she is pregnant, she should obtain a pregnancy test immediately and discuss with her physician whether she should continue taking Paxil or not. For a complete discussion on the effects of the drug during pregnancy, see the following section.

SAFETY OF USE DURING PREGNANCY

Paxil is classified under the Food and Drug Administration's Pregnancy Classification as Category C. Category C means animal studies have shown an adverse effect on an animal fetus. However, no one has conducted adequate studies in humans, but the benefits of taking the drug during pregnancy must truly outweigh the risks based on the results of animal testing. Animal studies using as much as nine to fifty times the maximum daily dose of Paxil showed no harm to the unborn fetus. When Paxil was given to rats in the third trimester of pregnancy, an increase in the number young dying in the first four days after birth was observed. It is important to know that extensive studies on the effect of Paxil on the human fetus is lacking. If you suspect that you are pregnant, contact your doctor immediately. The manufacturer strongly recommends that Paxil be used during pregnancy only if the benefits of taking the drug significantly outweigh the risks of potential harm to the fetus.

SAFETY OF USE WHEN BREAST-FEEDING

Paxil is excreted in the breast milk. The concentration of the drug in breast milk is similar to that found in the mother's bloodstream. Well-controlled studies regarding the effect on the infant of breast milk containing Paxil are lacking. Therefore, in the best interest of the infant, mothers should never breast-feed while taking the drug.

EXCRETION FROM THE BODY

Paxil is primarily metabolized by the liver and is removed from the body by the kidneys (64 percent) and the feces (36 percent) through the bowels. This process is very slow, which results in the drug staying in the body for quite some time. In fact, the drug will stay in the body for about twenty-four hours after taking a single dose and one to three days after several days of therapy with Paxil. The liver metabolizes Paxil into various inactive chemical compounds. These chemical compounds are only about one-fiftieth as active as Paxil in treating depression and OCD. Patients who have been taking the drug for several weeks should not expect the body to be free of the drug until about one week after taking the last dose.

WHAT TO KNOW BEFORE YOU USE THIS DRUG

Because the drug is metabolized by the liver, patients with liver disease, hepatitis, or cirrhosis may require lower doses. Physicians should make the same consideration for patients with kidney disease. Lower doses may be required in these patients as well. Also, patients who suffer from seizure disorders or epilepsy may want to inform their doctor of this condition before taking Paxil. The weight loss that occurs rarely when taking Paxil should be considered carefully. In some patients, this side effect may be undesirable. Paxil also causes a dry mouth (decrease in saliva flow) in some individuals. This may contribute to cavity formation and periodontal disease in a small number of individuals.

Paxil is not considered a "quick fix" in treating depression or OCD. The drug may require several weeks of therapy before a significant improvement is seen. Therefore, patients should not become discouraged and quit taking the drug if they do not see immediate improvement. The drug should be taken for at least four to six weeks before the patient and his or her physician decide the drug is not working and that some other medication should be used.

PROPER USE OF THE DRUG

Paxil should be taken every day in order to receive its maximum benefits. The patient should follow the dosing schedule set by his or her physician as closely as possible. Do not take more or less of the drug than is prescribed. Some patients may try to increase the dose on their own if they feel the drug is not effective at the prescribed dose. This may increase the risk of unwanted side effects and other adverse events. Other patients may try to decrease their dose on their own if they experience some unwanted side effects. This may result in too low of a dose being taken. Patients experiencing any unwanted side effects or who feel that the current dose may be too low should discuss this with their physician or pharmacist before adjusting the amount of medication.

If a patient forgets to take his or her daily dose and remembers within two to four hours of when the dose was to be taken, the patient should take the drug as soon as he or she remembers. If the patient forgets to take the daily dose and remembers more than four hours after the medication time, he or she should skip the missed dose and continue on the normal dosing schedule the next day or take the next scheduled dose on time. Patients should not double the dose.

IMPORTANT PATIENT INFORMATION

Individuals taking Paxil should make regular visits to their physician to check and discuss the progress of their condition. At that time, patients should report any side effects or other adverse effects to their physician. If a skin rash, itching, or hives occur after taking the drug, stop taking the drug and contact your physician as soon as possible. These may be the signs and symptoms of an allergic reaction to the drug. If these symptoms are accompanied by tightness in the chest or trouble breathing, seek medical attention immediately.

Paxil may cause some drowsiness and tiredness, especially at first. Based on clinical use and experience, Paxil tends to cause more drowsiness than Prozac or Luvox. The degree of drowsiness Paxil causes is less severe than that caused by pain killers, sleeping pills, and other nerve medications. Patients should use extreme caution when driving, operating heavy machinery or equipment, or doing jobs that require a great deal of mental alertness. Therefore, when taking the drug for the first few doses, patients should be cautious of its potential to cause drowsiness and observe how it affects them personally. The degree of drowsiness caused by the drug varies from patient to patient.

It is also important to know that alcohol, nerve medications, pain killers, muscle relaxers, antihistamines, allergy and cold medications, cough syrups, and other drugs known to cause drowsiness may significantly increase the drowsiness caused by Paxil. Therefore, extreme caution should be used when taking Paxil with these drugs. The drug may also cause some dizziness or lightheadedness, especially when getting up suddenly from lying or sitting positions.

Some patients taking Paxil may experience a dry mouth for a short period of time. This side effect is similar in severity to the dry mouth caused by some antihistamines. This side effect can be alleviated by chewing sugarless gum or candy. If the dry mouth continues for more than two weeks, patients should contact their physician.

If stomach upset or mild nausea occurs after taking Paxil, the patient may take it with food or milk to reduce this irritating side effect. If the nausea or stomach upset is severe, continues every time the drug is taken for several days, or vomiting occurs, contact your physician or pharmacist.

Most often Paxil is prescribed to be taken in the morning. Food, milk, and antacids do not significantly affect the action of the drug in the body or its absorption in the stomach. Therefore, the drug may be taken with breakfast or a morning snack.

STORAGE OF THE DRUG

Paxil, like all medications, should be kept out of the reach of children. Store the drug away from direct light and heat. Never store any medication in a bathroom medicine cabinet. Heat, moisture, and steam from the shower, bathtub, and sink may cause medications to become ineffective. Medications should also not be stored near the kitchen sink or in any other damp place for the same reasons. Ideally, your prescription medications should be stored in a tight, light-resistant (amber or brown) prescription bottle between 59 and 86 degrees and at no more than 104 degrees. Medications are best stored in the original bottles in which they were dispensed. Remember, the temperatures in a hot car or truck can exceed 105 degrees very easily. Therefore, medications should never be left in a hot car or truck for more than thirty to sixty minutes.

FURTHER INFORMATION

Individuals who would like further information on Paxil should first contact their pharmacist and then their physician. Another source of in-depth information is your local hospital. Many large hospitals, especially those associated with universities, have drug information centers. When calling the hospital, ask for the pharmacy department or drug information center of the hospital. Finally, individuals can contact the company that manufactures and markets the drug directly. SmithKline Beecham Pharmaceuticals, which manufactures Paxil, can be reached at this address: SmithKline Beecham Pharmaceuticals, ATT: Medical Department, One Franklin Plaza, P.O. Box 7929, Philadelphia, PA 19101. The phone number is (215) 751-5231 or (800) 366-8900.

FIVE

❧

Prozac

BRAND NAME

The brand name of the drug is Prozac.

GENERIC NAME

The generic name of the drug is fluoxetine. Currently no generic form is available. The patent on the drug expires in 2001. By this time, a generic alternative will probably be available.

DOSAGE FORMS

Prozac is available in 10mg and 20mg capsules and a 20mg-per-5ml mint-flavored liquid.

APPROVED AND ACCEPTED USES

The drug has been approved for use in adult patients with major depression. A major depression episode is defined as a persistent depressed mood that interferes with daily functioning nearly every day for at least two weeks. It should also include at least four of the following eight symptoms: change in appetite, change in sleep, loss of interest in usual activities, decreased sex drive, increased feeling of tiredness, feeling of guilt or worthlessness, slowed thinking or impaired concentration, and a suicide attempt or thoughts of suicide.

Prozac has also been approved for use in obsessive-compulsive disorder (OCD). OCD is defined as the obsessions or compulsions that cause extreme distress, are time-consuming, or significantly interfere with functioning socially or at work. The patient recognizes these behaviors as excessive and unreasonable, but still cannot control the urge to perform them.

Prozac has also recently been approved for bulimia nervosa and associated eating disorders. Prozac is used to treat the behavior of binge-eating and vomiting in patients with moderate to severe bulimia, which is defined as having at least three binge-eating/vomiting episodes per week for six months.

USUAL DOSE

The usual dose in treating depression is 20mg to 60mg daily. Researchers have conducted studies to test the effectiveness of 20mg, 40mg, and 80mg daily doses. Most studies indicate that 20mg once daily in the morning is usually enough to obtain the desired antidepressive effect. The physician may, however, increase the dose after several weeks if the patient sees no significant improvement in symptoms. Patients may take doses of 40mg or 80mg once a day in the morning or twice a day in the morning and at noon. Individuals should not take more than 80mg of Prozac per day. The drug may require several weeks of treatment before patients see noticeable improvement. Therefore, individuals should not expect immediate results or spontaneous miracle when taking the drug.

The usual dose in treating obsessive-compulsive disorder (OCD) is 20mg once daily in the morning. The doctor may prescribe higher doses of up to 80mg per day if, after several weeks of treatment with the 20mg dose, the patient sees no improvement. Patients may take doses higher than 20mg once daily in the morning or divided into two equal doses given in the morning and at noon. Unlike depression, higher doses of up to 80mg may be required in treating OCD. As with depression, individuals should not take more than 80mg of Prozac per day for OCD.

Dosages for treating bulimia are higher than for depression and OCD. The usual dose is 60mg once daily in the morning. Patients may start on a lower dose and slowly increase to the 60mg per day level under a doctor's supervision. The effectiveness in treating bulimia with doses higher than 60mg per day have not been studied. The maximum daily dose is 80mg.

ONSET OF ACTIVITY AND LENGTH OF ACTION

After a patient takes a single dose of Prozac, the drug stays in the body for approximately two to three days. After several days of use, the drug stays in the body approximately four to six days. It usually takes between one to four weeks before patients see noticeable improvement in symptoms. In some individuals the time period for improvement may be several weeks or even a few months. If the patient sees no improvement after several weeks, the physician may want to consider increasing the dose or switching the individual to another drug. Even though the drug is most often given for long periods of time, the effectiveness of long-term use has not been adequately studied.

CLINICAL TRIALS

The information on the effectiveness of Prozac in the manufacturer's clinical tests is presented here to demonstrate one major point. It's important to know that not all patients who take a drug will see an improvement in their symptoms. Just because the Food and Drug Administration (FDA) has approved a drug and determined it to be safe and effective doesn't mean that it works in every patient who takes it. In fact, for many drugs, the number of patients that actually benefit from the drug and see a significant improvement in their disease or symptoms may be as low as 50 percent. This is not to say that the results presented should discourage patients from taking or trying Prozac, but that the same drug may produce different results in different patients. The solution to this dilemma is for the physician to keep trying several different medications until he or she finds the most effective choice.

Major Depression

The manufacturer and other researchers investigated the effectiveness of Prozac in several clinical studies before the FDA approved the drug. Other similar clinical studies, conducted since FDA approval, have echoed many of the same results in treating depression. Prozac was shown to be significantly more effective than a placebo (a placebo is a pill with no medical properties) in improving the symptoms associated with a major depressive episode. Patients in these studies saw an improvement in their depressed mood, sleep disturbances, and in the amount of nervousness and anxiety experienced. A small number of patients, however, did not see an improvement in their depression.

Obsessive-Compulsive Disorder

For patients with obsessive-compulsive disorder (OCD), two clinical studies found that symptoms did improve. The manufacturer conducted these studies before the drug was approved to treat OCD. Other studies since that time have found similar results. The following table illustrates the results of study participants regarding their symptoms associated with OCD.

IMPROVEMENT IN SYMPTOMS ASSOCIATED WITH OCD

Outcome	No Drug	20mg Prozac	40mg Prozac	60mg Prozac
Worse	8%	0%	0%	0%
No change	65%	41%	33%	29%
Slightly improved	17%	23%	28%	24%
Much improved	8%	28%	27%	28%
Very much improved	3%	8%	12%	19%

As you can see in this study, patients did see some improvement in their symptoms associated with OCD. As the dose was increased, some patients saw even more improvement. This does not suggest, however, that higher doses should be used at the beginning of treatment. Physicians should always choose the lowest possible dose where the most improvement in symptoms is seen.

Bulimia

The effect of Prozac to treat bulimia was just recently studied by the manufacturer using both 20mg and 60mg daily doses. The 60mg daily dose produced significantly better results. In fact, patients saw noticeable improvement as early as one week after beginning treatment with Prozac. Some patients experienced a complete disappearance of the binge-eating/vomiting behaviors. Most patients, however, saw only a reduction in the number of binge-eating/vomiting episodes. These results indicate that the drug is not a wonder-drug cure for bulimia, but it does improve and lessen the severity of the condition. Again, some bulimic patients did not see any improvement in symptoms when taking Prozac.

CONTRAINDICATIONS

Prozac is metabolized by the liver. This means that patients with liver diseases, such as cirrhosis and hepatitis, should possibly take a lower dose and take the drug less often. Patients with severe liver disease may want to be treated with a drug that is metabolized and excreted exclusively by the kidneys instead. Individuals with liver problems or disorders should discuss this with their doctor before taking Prozac.

Patients with kidney disease should follow the same precautions as those with liver disease. Even though the drug is primarily metabolized by the liver, individuals with severe kidney problems may require smaller doses of Prozac and those doses may be given less often. Again, individuals with kidney problems or disorders should discuss these issues with their doctor before taking Prozac.

There have been reports of serious and sometimes fatal reactions in patients taking Prozac and MAO inhibitors such as Eldepryl, Furoxone, Matulane, Nardil, and Parnate. Some of these reactions include high body temperature, rapid fluctuations of vital signs (high blood pressure and fast heartbeat), changes in mental status, extreme agitation, delirious behavior, and even coma. Some of these reactions have occurred as long as five weeks between the use of Prozac and the other drugs. Therefore, Prozac therapy should not be started until at least five weeks after the patient has stopped taking one of these drugs. If the patient has been using Prozac for long periods of time (greater than three months), he or she should not start therapy with Eldepryl, Furoxone, Matulane, Nardil, or Parnate until at least five to seven weeks after Prozac has been stopped.

WARNINGS AND PRECAUTIONS

Prozac may cause some adverse effects that may be bothersome to some patients. The adverse effects that warrant special consideration usually occur in only a small number of individuals, but the seriousness of their consequences affords them special consideration and explanation. These effects are not included to frighten patients, but more importantly to give them vital information based on the experiences of other patients.

In some clinical testing of Prozac for depression, 12 percent to 16 percent of patients experienced anxiety, nervousness, or insomnia. In clinical testing for OCD, 28 percent of patients reported insomnia and 14 percent reported nervousness or anxiety. In other clinical trials for bulimia, 33 percent reported insomnia, 15 percent reported anxiety, and 11 percent reported nervousness. These adverse effects may aggravate or be bothersome to some individuals suffering from these conditions.

Significant weight loss and loss of appetite, especially in underweight depressed or bulimic patients, has occurred in patients taking Prozac. This effect may be undesirable in some patients. In clinical trials for depression, 11 percent experienced some loss of appetite and 2 percent of patients experienced significant weight loss. In clinical trials for OCD, 17 percent experienced loss of appetite. And in clinical trials for bulimia, 8 percent experienced loss of appetite.

A significant problem discovered during the manufacturer's clinical testing was the occurrence of manic episodes. These episodes were very rare. In fact, less than 1 percent of patients taking the drug experienced a manic-type episode. Another problem was that a small number of patients experienced seizures or convulsions. Approximately 0.1 percent of patients experienced a seizure while taking Prozac. This percentage seems to be similar to the effects of other antidepressants and could not definitely be linked to Prozac. It is, however, important for patients with epilepsy or other seizure disorders to be cautious when using Prozac. No studies to date have examined the potential of the drug to increase the number of seizures in patients with epilepsy or other seizure disorders.

A lot of media attention has focused on Prozac's purported ability to increase suicidal tendencies or drive patients to commit suicide. It must be noted that suicidal thoughts are one of the primary symptoms of depression. It is hard to determine if it is the drug itself or the depressive episode that is the cause for suicidal thoughts and attempts. Until further studies can be conducted to determine the potential for Prozac to cause suicide, the conclusions about the increased risk of suicide while taking the drug are questionable.

The manufacturer of Prozac does, however, recommend close supervision of high-risk patients when beginning therapy with Prozac. These same precautions are suggested when treating patients with OCD as well as bulimia.

Clinical experience in patients with other chronic diseases who take Prozac is limited. It is known that none of the patients taking the drug experienced any cardiac problems as measured by an electrocardiogram. The average heart rate of study participants, however, decreased by three beats per minute in clinical trials.

USE IN THE ELDERLY

The use of Prozac in elderly patients (sixty years and older) with depression has been studied. The drug was found to be effective in treating depression in this group of patients. Currently, no reduction in dose is necessary in elderly individuals who are reasonably healthy. However, older patients with serious medical conditions or those on multiple medications should discuss this with their doctor. These conditions may require smaller or less frequent doses of Prozac.

USE IN CHILDREN

Prozac is currently not approved for use in children. This does not mean, however, that physicians are not prescribing the drug for children. For a complete discussion on the use of Prozac and other SSRIs in children, refer to Chapter 8, "Children and SSRIs."

AVERAGE RETAIL PRICES

The prices listed here are for informational purposes only. I presented them to provide some basic information regarding the approximate cost of the drug Prozac. These prices are averages and may vary from pharmacy to pharmacy or within different regions of the country.

As is the case with some other prescription drugs, you might expect that the larger the dose, the larger the cost. Example: A 20mg capsule theoretically should cost twice as much as a 10mg capsule. For this particular class of drugs, the SSRIs, this is not the case. All three strengths of the drug cost the pharmacy approximately the same (within ten to twenty dollars per one hundred tablets) no matter what the strength. Therefore, prices for the 10mg and 20mg capsules may be somewhat similar.

Drug and Strength	Quantity	Retail Price
Prozac 10mg	30 capsules	$70.99–$91.49
Prozac 20mg	30 capsules	$71.69–$92.50
Prozac 20mg/5ml	4 ounces (120ml)	$103.00–$153.49

SIDE EFFECTS

The side effects listed below were discovered during well-controlled clinical trials before the FDA approved the drug for use. Researchers believe the occurrence of these side effects under the drug's normal everyday use in real world settings to be very similar. Side effects are listed in decreasing order based on the percentage of patients experiencing certain side effects. The percentages listed below are averages based on several different clinical tests and are believed to be reliable.

Side Effect	Percentage Experiencing
Nausea/upset stomach	23%
Headache	21%
Insomnia	20%
Nervousness	13%
Anxiety	13%
Drowsiness	13%
Diarrhea	12%
Weakness/loss of strength	12%
Loss of appetite	11%
Dizziness	10%
Tremors	10%
Dry mouth	10%
Indigestion	8%
Increased sweating	8%

Side Effect	Percentage Experiencing
Flulike symptoms	5%
Pharyngitis	5%
Decreased sex drive	4%
Rash	4%
Itching	3%
Low blood pressure	3%
Gas	3%
Vomiting	3%
Increased yawning	3%
Abnormal vision	3%
Weight loss	2%
Fever	2%
Pounding heartbeat	2%

The side effects listed above were reported by patients and, for the most part, were mild to moderate in severity. In fact, only 1 percent to 2 percent of the patients experiencing insomnia, nervousness, or anxiety felt these side effects were bothersome enough to stop taking Prozac.

Researchers also discovered other side effects during clinical testing. These side effects occurred in a very small number of patients who had taken Prozac. Some of these side effects are very serious; it's important to remember, however, that only a very small number of patients taking Prozac even experienced these side effects. This should not discourage patients in any way from taking the drug Prozac. Many prescription drugs have most of these same side effects that occur infrequently or rarely with their use.

These side effects occurred infrequently (0.1 percent to 1 percent) in patients taking Prozac. (Note: 1 percent = 1 in every 100 patients and 0.1 percent = 1 in every 1,000 patients.)

chills

swelling of the face

pelvic pain

low body temperature

feeling bad or not well

chest pains

irregular heartbeat

congestive heart failure

fast heartbeat

migraine

colitis

bleeding gums

increased salivation

taste changes

abnormal liver tests

skin discoloration

sores in the mouth

stomach ulcer

increased thirst

decreased activity of the
   thyroid gland

anemia

dehydration

swelling

gout

high cholesterol

euphoria

hallucinations

abnormal dreams

bone pain

muscle pain

arthritic bursitis

increased sex drive

psychosis

personality disorders

asthma

bloody nose

increased hiccups

acne

hair loss

abnormal menstrual period

breast pain

breast milk production

urinary problems

dry eyes

ringing in the ears

increased sensitivity of the
   eyes to sunlight

The following list of side effects occurred very rarely (0.001 percent to 0.1 percent or less) in patients taking Prozac. (Note: 0.1 percent = 1 in every 1,000 patients and 0.001 percent = 1 in every 100,000 patients.)

increased sensitivity of the
   skin to sunburn

low body temperature

slow heartbeat

embolism in the brain

shock

inflammation of the veins in
   the leg

gallbladder pain

bloody diarrhea

intestinal ulcer

hepatitis

intestinal obstruction
swelling of the tongue
blood disorders
purplish-red blotches on the skin
diabetes
alcohol intolerance
low calcium and iron
increased potassium
muscle weakness
antisocial reactions
delusions
decreased reflexes
trouble breathing
cough
swelling in the lungs
psoriasis
hearing problems
loss of taste
vision problems
kidney pain

These side effects are presented for information purposes only, not to scare individuals currently taking Prozac or to prevent them from taking it in the future. My hope is to increase the patient's awareness, and to report that in some rare instances the drug has caused serious side effects. Prozac and the SSRIs in general are some of the safest drugs on the market used to treat depression and OCD. However, you should discuss any abnormal side effects that you experience while taking Prozac with your physician and pharmacist.

DRUG INTERACTIONS

Compared with other drugs used to treat depression and OCD, Prozac and the SSRIs in general have fewer drug interactions. A drug interaction occurs when two drugs taken together produce an unwanted side effect or adverse effect, or when they affect how one drug or the other works in the body that is different from its intended use. The five drug interactions listed below are the most clinically significant and potentially the most serious.

1. Prozac should never be taken with Eldepryl, Furoxone, Matulane, Nardil, or Parnate. This can cause a very serious and potentially life-threatening

condition called serotonin syndrome. Symptoms of serotonin syndrome include mental status changes, confusion, restlessness, shivering, tremor, diarrhea, agitation, severe convulsions, and very high blood pressure. If serotonin syndrome is recognized early enough, the patient usually recovers quickly once these drugs are discontinued. However, there have been deaths associated with this lethal combination. Physicians administer no actual treatment for serotonin syndrome, except for supportive care of body functions (maintaining adequate blood pressure, heart function, breathing, etc.).

Patients taking Prozac should not take Eldepryl, Furoxone, Matulane, Nardil, or Parnate until at least five weeks after discontinuing treatment with Prozac. Conversely, patients who have taken Eldepryl, Furoxone, Matulane, Nardil, or Parnate should not be started on Prozac until at least five weeks after any of these drugs has been discontinued.

2. Prozac may significantly increase the drowsiness or sleepiness caused by alcohol, nerve medications, pain killers, muscle relaxers, antihistamines, allergy medications, cold medications, and cough syrups. This may be dangerous when driving, operating heavy machinery, or during any other task requiring mental alertness. This is not to say patients cannot take Prozac and these other drugs together. Patients just need to be aware that a significant increase in drowsiness may occur.

3. Prozac may increase the blood levels of Lanoxin or Coumadin. This may lead to increased bleeding in patients taking Coumadin, which may be very serious, especially when patients first start taking Prozac or have recently discontinued it. This interaction may require your physician to adjust the dosage of Coumadin. Once the Coumadin dosage

is stabilized, patients can take Coumadin and Prozac safely together.

The effect of Prozac on Lanoxin is not as severe, and complications are not as common. Patients taking Lanoxin should, however, discuss this with their physician before taking Prozac.

4. Prozac may increase the blood levels of Dilantin, which may produce toxic symptoms. Patients taking Prozac should have their physician measure and assess their blood levels of Dilantin. Dosage adjustments of Dilantin may be required when taken with Prozac. However, if a physician closely monitors Dilantin blood levels, Prozac and Dilantin can be taken together.

5. The amino acid tryptophan, contained in some vitamin supplements, should not be taken in large amounts with Prozac. Tryptophan is one of the chemicals that serotonin is made from in the body. SSRIs like Prozac increase the amount of serotonin available in the body. If a patient takes an excessive amount of tryptophan, the body may produce more serotonin than normal. This overproduction along with Prozac's effect on serotonin can result in excessive serotonin levels. This may cause agitation, restlessness, insomnia, anxiety, and stomach problems like nausea, vomiting, and diarrhea. Therefore, vitamin supplements with large amounts of tryptophan should be avoided.

Other potential drug interactions are also worth mentioning. These interactions do not occur as frequently as the others listed above and are not nearly as serious.

1. Prozac may increase the blood levels of Anafranil, Asendin, Desyrel, Elavil, Limbitrol, Ludiomil, Norpramin, Pamelor, Sinequan, Surmontil, Tofranil, and Vivactil. This interaction may increase the side effects of these drugs.

2. Prozac may increase the blood levels of Valium and Xanax in some patients. This may lead to increased side effects associated with taking Valium or Xanax such as drowsiness, confusion, and lack of mental alertness.

3. Prozac may increase the amount and severity of side effects of the following drugs: Compazine, Etrafon, Haldol, Loxitane, Mellaril, Moban, Navane, Orap, Prolixin, Serentil, Stelazine, Thorazine, and Trilafon.

4. Prozac may alter the blood levels of lithium, which may lead to toxic effects. Blood levels of lithium should be measured and monitored.

5. Recently, there have been rare reports of Prozac causing weakness, muscle reflex problems, and coordination problems when taken with Imitrex. Individuals should be aware of this potential drug interaction and use caution when taking Prozac and Imitrex together.

FOOD INTERACTIONS

Prozac may be taken with or without food or milk. Food does not affect the amount of drug absorbed from the stomach and intestines. In fact, individuals who experience mild nausea when taking the drug on an empty stomach may take it with food or milk.

DEALING WITH OVERDOSES

It is possible to overdose on Prozac when taking large quantities alone or with other drugs and/or alcohol. The main symptoms of overdose are nausea and vomiting. Other symptoms of an overdose include agitation, nervousness, and restlessness. Deaths have been associated with overdose, but these occurred when patients took large quantities of Prozac (greater than 1000mg) and are extremely rare. If you suspect that you or someone else has taken an overdose of Prozac, contact your nearest poison control center immediately.

ALLERGIES

Individuals who have a past history of being allergic to Prozac should not take the drug. Individuals allergic to other similar drugs in the same class, such as Zoloft, Paxil, or Luvox, should alert their doctor of this and use caution when taking Prozac. In U.S. clinical trials, 7 percent of the patients tested exhibited some form of allergic reaction to Prozac. Most of the patients who experienced an allergic reaction reported only itching and a skin rash. However, some patients also reported fever, carpal tunnel syndrome, swollen glands, muscle pain, swelling, and/or trouble breathing. These symptoms disappeared in most patients once the drug was discontinued or when patients were treated with antihistamines and/or steroids. If a rash, itching, swelling, fever, or swollen glands occurs while you are taking Prozac, contact your doctor. If chest pain, difficulty in breathing, or the other symptoms listed above become worse, seek emergency medical treatment as quickly as possible.

CANCER-CAUSING POTENTIAL

There is no evidence that Prozac has the potential to cause cancer at this time, even at very high doses. Studies have been conducted on rats that were given doses five to nine times the maximum human dose of 80mg. These studies showed no evidence of the drug causing cancer. However, no one has conducted any well-controlled studies in humans. But cancer-causing studies on rats usually are good predictors of the likely effects in humans regarding cancer-causing potential.

EFFECT ON SEXUAL FUNCTION

There is no concrete evidence that Prozac has any effect on sexual function, including the ability to have an orgasm, the ability to maintain an erection, the ability to ejaculate, or the ability to enjoy sex in general. There was, however, a slightly decreased effect on sexual desire.

EFFECT ON FERTILITY

There is no evidence that Prozac will cause fertility problems in either men or women. It is, however, important to realize that risks are associated with taking any drug if a woman believes she is pregnant. If a woman suspects she is pregnant, she should obtain a pregnancy test immediately and discuss with her physician whether she should continue taking Prozac or not. For a complete discussion on the effects of the drug during pregnancy, see the following section.

SAFETY OF USE DURING PREGNANCY

Prozac is classified under the Food and Drug Administration's Pregnancy Classification as Category B. This means that no current evidence of risk in humans exists. Animal studies using as much as eleven times the maximum daily dose of Prozac (80mg) showed no harm to the unborn fetus. During clinical studies of the drug, seventeen women became pregnant accidentally. No complications, birth defects, or adverse effects were observed in the children of these seventeen women. Several small studies of women taking Prozac while pregnant also support the findings of no harm to the fetus.

However, one study did find a very slight increase in the number of spontaneous abortions and miscarriages. It is important to know that we lack extensive studies on the effect of the drug on the fetus. If you suspect that you are pregnant, contact your doctor immediately. Even though the risk of birth defects appears to be low, the benefits of taking the drug should be weighed against the potential risks.

Researchers almost never conduct tests of how a drug affects the fetus in pregnant women. However, a study assessing the effect on the fetus in women taking Prozac was published in the October 3, 1996, issue of the *New England Journal of Medicine* by Chambers et al. The study found that women treated with Prozac did not have a higher rate of spontaneous abortion or major abnormalities when compared to women who did not take the drug. However, women taking Prozac did have a higher rate of minor abnormalities in the fetus. The study also found that women who took Prozac in the third trimester (last three months) of pregnancy had higher rates of premature delivery, higher number of admissions to special-care nurseries, and more respiratory difficulty; their babies had lower birth weight and shorter overall length. The study concluded that the greatest risk to the fetus of women taking Prozac is in the third trimester of pregnancy. However, caution should be used by women during their entire pregnancy.

SAFETY OF USE WHEN BREAST-FEEDING

Prozac is excreted in the breast milk. Therefore, women taking Prozac should not breast-feed. In some limited case studies, no adverse effects were reported in a breast-fed infant whose mother was taking Prozac. Another case study, however, found that one infant developed crying spells, problems sleeping, vomiting, and watery diarrhea. These cases are isolated incidents. We lack well-controlled studies regarding how breast milk containing Prozac affects infants. Therefore, in the best interest of the infant, mothers should never breast-feed while taking the drug.

EXCRETION FROM THE BODY

Prozac is primarily metabolized by the liver and removed from the body by the kidneys. This process is very slow and results in the drug staying in the body for quite some time. In fact, the drug will stay in the body for one to three days after taking a single dose and four to six days after several days of therapy with Prozac. Prozac is metabolized by the liver into the chemical norfluoxetine. This compound also provides a great deal of activity in treating depression, OCD, and Bulimia. The metabolite norfluoxetine is considered an active drug just like Prozac itself. Norfluoxetine will stay in the body anywhere from 4 to 16 days depending on how long Prozac has been taken. Patients who have taken a single dose of Prozac therefore should not expect the body to be free of the drug and its active metabolite for at least 7 to 10 days. Patients who have been taking the drug for several weeks should not expect the body to be free of the drug for up to 2 to 6 weeks.

WHAT TO KNOW BEFORE YOU USE THIS DRUG

Patients who are diabetic should note this when discussing taking Prozac with their physician. Prozac may affect blood sugar and require adjustments to insulin dosages. Because the drug is metabolized by the liver, patients with liver disease, hepatitis, or cirrhosis may require lower doses. Physicians should make the same consideration for patients with kidney disease. These patients may require lower doses as well. Also, patients who suffer from seizure disorders or epilepsy should inform their doctor of this before taking Prozac.

Prozac is not considered a "quick fix" in treating depression, OCD, or bulimia. The drug may require several weeks of therapy before patients see significant improvement. Therefore, patients should not become discouraged if immediate improvements are not seen and give up on taking the drug. The drug should be taken for at least 3–6 weeks before the patient and his/her physician decide the drug is not working and that some other medication should be used.

PROPER USE OF THE DRUG

Prozac should be taken every day in order to receive its maximum benefits. The patient should follow the dosing schedule set by his or her physician as closely as possible. Do not take more or less of the drug than is prescribed. Some patients may try to increase the dose on their own if they feel the drug is not effective at the prescribed dose. This may increase the risk of unwanted side effects and other adverse events. Other patients may try to decrease their dose on their own if they experience some unwanted side effects. This may result in too low of a dose being taken. Patients experiencing any unwanted side effects or who feel the current dose may be too low should discuss this with their physician or pharmacist before adjusting the amount of medication.

If a patient forgets to take his or her daily dose and remembers within two to four hours of when the dose was to be taken, the patient should take the drug as soon as he or she remembers. If the patient forgets to take the daily dose and remembers more than four hours after the medication time, he or she should skip the missed dose and continue on the normal dosing schedule the next day, or whenever the next dose is scheduled. Patients should not double the dose.

IMPORTANT PATIENT INFORMATION

Individuals taking Prozac should make regular visits to their physician to check and discuss the progress of their condition. At that time, patients should report any side effects or other adverse effects to their physician. If a skin rash, itching, or hives occur after taking the drug, stop taking the drug and contact your physician as soon as possible. These may be the signs and symptoms of an allergic reaction. In clinical trials of the drug involving 10,782 patients, about 7 percent experienced some form of an allergic reaction. If these symptoms are accompanied by tightness in the chest or trouble breathing, seek medical attention immediately.

Prozac may cause some drowsiness and tiredness, especially at first. The degree of drowsiness Prozac causes is less than that caused by pain killers, sleeping pills, and other nerve medications. Caution should be used when driving, operating heavy machinery or equipment, or doing jobs that require a great deal of mental alertness. Therefore, when taking the drug for the first few doses, patients should be cautious of its potential to cause drowsiness and observe how it affects them personally. The degree of drowsiness caused by the drug varies from patient to patient.

It is also important to know that alcohol, nerve medications, pain killers, muscle relaxers, antihistamines, allergy and cold medications, cough syrups, and other drugs known to cause drowsiness may significantly increase the drowsiness caused by Prozac. Therefore, extreme caution should be used when taking Prozac with these drugs. Prozac may also cause some limited dizziness or lightheadedness, especially when getting up suddenly from lying or sitting positions.

In a limited number of patients, Prozac may cause a dry mouth for a short period of time. This side effect is similar in severity to the dry mouth caused by some antihistamines. This side effect can be alleviated by chewing sugarless gum or candy. If the dry mouth continues for more than two weeks, contact your physician.

If stomach upset or mild nausea occurs after taking Prozac, the patient may take it with food or milk to reduce this irritating side effect. If the nausea or stomach upset is severe, continues every time the drug is taken for several days, or vomiting occurs, contact your physician or pharmacist.

Many times Prozac is prescribed to be taken in the morning. Food and milk do not affect the action of the drug in the body or its absorption in the stomach. Therefore, the drug may be taken with breakfast or morning snack.

STORAGE OF THE DRUG

Prozac, like all medications, should be kept out of the reach of children. Store the drug away from direct light and heat. Never store any medication in a bathroom medicine cabinet. Heat, moisture, and steam from the shower, bathtub, and sink may cause medications to become ineffective. Medications also should not be stored near the kitchen sink or in any other damp place for the same reason. Ideally, your prescription medications should be stored in a tight, light-resistant (amber or brown) prescription bottle between 59 and 86 degrees and at no more than 104 degrees. Medications are best stored in the original bottles in which they were dispensed. Remember, the temperatures in a hot car or truck can exceed 105 degrees very easily. Therefore, medications should never be left in a hot car or truck for more than thirty to sixty minutes.

FURTHER INFORMATION

Individuals who would like further information on Prozac should first contact their pharmacist and then their physician. Another source of in-depth information is your local hospital. Many large hospitals, especially those associated with universities, have drug information centers. When calling the hospital, ask for the pharmacy department or drug information center of the hospital. Finally, individuals can contact the company that manufactures and markets the drug directly. Prozac is manufactured by Eli Lilly and Co. and marketed by Dista Products Co., a marketing subsidiary of Eli Lilly and Co. Their address is: Dista Product Co., Lilly Research Laboratories, ATT: Medical Information, Lilly Corporate Center, Indianapolis, IN 46285. The phone number is (800) 545-5979.

SIX

❧

Zoloft

BRAND NAME

The brand name of the drug is Zoloft.

GENERIC NAME

The generic name of the drug is sertraline. Currently no generic form is available. The patent on the drug expires in 2005. By this time, a generic alternative will probably be available.

DOSAGE FORMS

Zoloft is available in 25mg, 50mg, and 100mg tablets. The drug is currently not available in a liquid form.

APPROVED AND ACCEPTED USES

Zoloft has been approved for use in adult patients with major depression. A major depression episode is defined as a persistent depressed mood that interferes with daily functioning nearly every day for at least two weeks. It should also include at least four of the following eight symptoms: change in appetite, change in sleep, loss of interest in usual activities, decreased sex drive, increased feeling of tiredness, feeling of guilt or worthlessness, slowed thinking or impaired concentration, and a suicide attempt or thoughts of suicide.

Zoloft has also been approved for use in obsessive-compulsive disorder (OCD). OCD is defined as obsessions or compulsions that cause extreme distress, are time-consuming, or significantly interfere with functioning socially or at work. The patient recognizes these behaviors as excessive and unreasonable, but still cannot control the urge to perform them.

Zoloft has also been approved for use in panic disorder. This may or may not include symptoms of agoraphobia (the fear of being in open or public places). Panic disorder is characterized by the occurrence of unexpected and recurrent panic attacks. Panic attacks usually have a discrete period of intense fear or discomfort that develops abruptly and reaches a peak within ten minutes. During this time, there is a sudden feeling of intense apprehension, fearfulness, terror, and/or impending doom. Panic attacks usually also include at least four or more of the following symptoms:

1. pounding heartbeat or increased heart rate
2. intense sweating
3. trembling or shaking
4. sensations of shortness of breath or feeling smothered
5. feeling of choking
6. chest pain or discomfort
7. nausea or stomach distress
8. feeling dizzy, unsteady, lightheaded, or faint
9. feelings of unreality or being detached from oneself
10. fear of losing control

11. fear of dying
12. numbness or tingling sensations
13. chills or hot flashes

These attacks may also include the associated concern about having additional attacks, worrying about the implications or consequences of the attacks, and/or a significant change in behavior related to the attacks.

USUAL DOSE

The usual dose in treating depression is 50mg to 200mg daily. Researchers have conducted studies to test the effectiveness of 50mg, 100mg, and 200mg daily doses. Most patients are started on a 50mg daily dose. In severe cases, patients may need doses as high as 100mg or 200mg per day in order to obtain the desired antidepressive effect. The physician may increase the Zoloft dosage to a maximum of 200mg per day after several weeks if the patient sees no significant improvement of the symptoms. Physicians should wait at least one to two weeks between dosage increases. Individuals should not take more than 200mg of Zoloft per day. The drug may require several weeks of treatment before patients see noticeable improvement. Therefore, individuals should not expect immediate results or a spontaneous miracle when taking the drug.

The usual dose in treating obsessive-compulsive disorder (OCD) is 50mg to 100mg once daily. The doctor may prescribe higher doses of up to 200mg per day if, after several weeks of treatment with the 50mg or 100mg dose, the patients see no improvement. As with depression, individuals should not take more than 200mg of Zoloft per day for OCD.

The usual dose in treating panic disorder is 25mg per day for the first week and then increased to 50mg daily thereafter. Patients may take higher doses of up to 200mg per day, depending on the patient's responsiveness. The maximum daily dose of Zoloft used to treat panic disorder should be no more than 200mg per day.

ONSET OF ACTIVITY AND LENGTH OF ACTION

After a patient takes a single dose of Zoloft, the drug stays in the body for approximately twenty-four hours. After several days of use, the drug stays in the body approximately forty-eight hours. It usually takes between two to four weeks before patients see a noticeable improvement in symptoms. In some individuals the time period for improvement may be several weeks or even a few months. If a patient sees no improvement after several weeks, the physician may want to consider increasing the dose or switching the individual to another drug. Even though the drug is most often given for long periods of time, the effectiveness of long-term use has not been adequately studied.

CLINICAL TRIALS

The information on the effectiveness of Zoloft in the manufacturer's clinical tests is presented here to demonstrate one major point. It's important to know that not all patients who take a drug will see an improvement in their symptoms. Just because the Food and Drug Administration (FDA) has approved a drug and determined it to be safe and effective doesn't mean that it works in every patient who takes it. In fact, for many drugs, the number of patients that actually benefit from the drug and see a significant improvement in their disease or symptoms may be as low as 50 percent. This is not to say that the results presented should discourage patients from taking or trying Zoloft, but that the same drug may produce different results in different patients. The solution to this dilemma is for the physician to keep trying several different medications until he or she finds the most effective choice.

Major Depression

The manufacturer investigated the effectiveness of Zoloft in several clinical studies before the FDA approved the drug for public use. Other similar clinical studies, conducted since FDA approval, have echoed many of the same results in treating depression. Zoloft was shown to be significantly superior to a placebo (a placebo is defined as a pill with no medical properties) in improving the symptoms associated with major depressive illnesses. Patients in these studies saw an improvement in their depressed mood, as well as an improvement in the other symptoms associated with depression. However, a small number of patients did not see an improvement in their depression.

Researchers studied a comparison of the effectiveness of several different doses (50mg, 100mg, 150mg, and 200mg) in treating depression. The study could not determine which particular dose was more effective in treating depression. This means that a physician must determine the most effective dose for each patient individually. Some patients may respond very well to a 50mg daily dose while others may require a dose as high as 200mg. There is no magic dose in treating depression with Zoloft.

Obsessive-Compulsive Disorder

When patients took Zoloft to treat obsessive-compulsive disorder (OCD), three clinical studies found that symptoms did improve. The manufacturer conducted these studies after the FDA approved the drug for use in treating depression. All three studies found that Zoloft was responsible for a significant improvement in the symptoms associated with OCD. Differences in age and gender (male versus female) were also studied. Researchers found Zoloft to be effective in treating OCD regardless of age or gender. Other studies since that time have found similar results regarding effectiveness in treating OCD.

The OCD clinical studies used slightly higher doses compared to the depression clinical studies. This does not suggest, however, that physicians should prescribe higher doses at the beginning of treatment with Zoloft. But higher doses may be required to effectively treat OCD as compared with depression. However, physicians should always choose the lowest possible dose where the most improvement in symptoms is seen.

Panic Disorder

Three large ten- to twelve-week clinical studies demonstrated the effectiveness of Zoloft in treating panic disorder. In these studies, Zoloft was significantly more effective than a placebo (inert pill) in reducing the frequency of panic attacks. On average, patients taking Zoloft had two fewer panic attacks per week as compared to those patients who did not receive the drug. Patients taking Zoloft also reported themselves as significantly more improved as compared to patients taking a placebo in overall quality of life.

CONTRAINDICATIONS

Zoloft is metabolized by the liver. This means that patients with liver diseases, even mild or stable cirrhosis or hepatitis, should take a lower dose and/or take the drug less often. Patients with severe liver disease may want to be treated with a drug that is metabolized and excreted exclusively by the kidneys instead. Studies have been conducted with patients who have liver disease and who have been given Zoloft. In patients with liver disease, the drug stayed in the body twice as long and blood concentrations increased significantly. Therefore, individuals with liver problems or disorders should discuss this with their doctor before taking Zoloft.

Patients with kidney disease should follow the same precautions as those with liver disease. Even though the drug is primarily metabolized by the liver, individuals with severe kidney problems may require smaller doses of Zoloft and may need to take those doses less often. The effects of Zoloft in patients with kidney disease or those who require renal dialysis have not been studied. Therefore, individuals with kidney problems or disorders should discuss these issues with their doctor before taking Zoloft.

There have been reports of serious and even fatal reactions in patients taking Zoloft and MAO inhibitors such as Eldepryl, Furoxone, Matulane, Nardil, and Parnate. Some of these reactions have included high body temperature, rapid fluctuations of vital signs (high blood pressure and fast heartbeat), changes in mental status, extreme agitation, delirious behavior, and even coma. Some of these reactions have occurred as long as two weeks between the use of Zoloft and Eldepryl, Furoxone, Matulane, Nardil, or Parnate. Therefore, Zoloft therapy should not be started until at least two weeks after the patient has stopped taking the MAO inhibitors. If the patient has been using Zoloft for long periods of time (greater than three months), he or she should not start therapy with these drugs until at least two to three weeks after treatment with Zoloft has been stopped.

WARNINGS AND PRECAUTIONS

Zoloft may cause adverse effects that may be bothersome to some patients. The adverse effects that warrant special consideration usually occur in only a small number of individuals, but the seriousness of their consequences affords them special consideration and explanation. These side effects are not included in this book to frighten people taking Zoloft, but more importantly to give them vital information based on the experiences of other patients.

In some clinical testing of Zoloft for depression, 0.4 percent of patients (4 in 1,000 patients) experienced hypomania or mania. This adverse effect may aggravate or be bothersome to some individuals suffering from these conditions. Physicians should especially monitor patients who are diagnosed as bipolar or manic-depressive.

A small amount of weight loss and loss of appetite have occurred in patients taking Zoloft. The weight loss associated with taking Zoloft was only 1 to 2 pounds. This effect, however, may be undesirable in some patients. Only very rarely have patients stopped taking Zoloft because of weight loss or loss of appetite.

Physicians should also take precautions for those patients who have experienced seizures or convulsions. The effect of Zoloft on the frequency, duration, and severity of seizures and convulsions has not been extensively studied. No studies to date have examined the potential of the drug to increase the number of seizures in patients with epilepsy or other seizure disorders. However, in clinical trials for OCD, 4 patients out of 1,800 experienced seizures. In clinical trials for depression involving 3,000 patients, none of the patients experienced seizures. The higher number of patients experiencing seizures in the OCD trials versus the depression trials may be because higher doses of the drug were typically used in treating OCD. Therefore, patients on high doses of Zoloft may be slightly more likely to experience a seizure. It is important to consider that other medications similar to Zoloft have been known to cause seizures or convulsions in a small number of patients. Therefore, patients with epilepsy or a history of seizures or convulsions should be cautious when using Zoloft.

A lot of media attention has focused on Prozac's purported ability to increase suicidal tendencies or drive patients to commit suicide. Patients therefore may wonder if taking Zoloft may cause the same suicidal tendencies because the two drugs are similar. Suicidal thoughts are one of the primary symptoms of depression, so it is hard to determine if it is the drug itself or the depressive episode that is causing suicidal thoughts and attempts. Until further studies can be conducted to determine the potential for Prozac or Zoloft to cause suicidal thoughts, the conclusions about the increased risk of suicide while taking these drugs are questionable.

The manufacturer of Prozac does, however, recommend close supervision of high-risk patients when beginning therapy with Prozac. These same considerations should also be given to patients taking Zoloft.

Clinical experience in patients with other chronic diseases and who take Zoloft is limited. Caution is required, however, in individuals with metabolic or blood disorders. There have been rare reports of altered platelet function in patients taking Zoloft. These reports include patients experiencing abnormal bleeding and purple spots on the skin, indicating broken blood vessels beneath the skin. Whether Zoloft was solely responsible for these adverse effects was not clear.

Zoloft has not been studied in patients with heart disease or who have suffered a heart attack. However, electrocardiograms (ECGs) in healthy individuals taking Zoloft were normal (they did not show any significant abnormalities). Several cases of excessive sodium loss from the body or low sodium levels have occurred in patients taking Zoloft. This condition is known as hyponatremia, a condition, like other electrolyte disturbances such as low potassium, that may be serious, especially in the elderly. The majority of these cases occurred in the elderly, with a few cases occurring in patients taking diuretics (water pills). The hyponatremia caused by Zoloft is usually reversible once the drug is discontinued.

USE IN THE ELDERLY

The use of Zoloft in the elderly (patients sixty years and older) with depression has been studied. The drug was found to be effective in treating depression in this group of patients. Currently, no reduction in dose is necessary in elderly individuals who are reasonably healthy. However, older patients with serious medical conditions or those on multiple medications should discuss this with their doctor. These conditions may require smaller or less frequent doses of Zoloft.

USE IN CHILDREN

Zoloft is currently not approved for use in children. This does not mean, however, that physicians are not prescribing the drug for children. The manufacturer has not conducted any well-controlled studies regarding Zoloft's use in children. For a complete discussion on the use of Zoloft and other SSRIs in children, refer to Chapter 8, "Children and SSRIs."

AVERAGE RETAIL PRICES

The prices listed here are for informational purposes only. I present them to provide some basic information regarding the approximate cost of the drug Zoloft. These prices are averages and may vary from pharmacy to pharmacy or within different regions of the country.

As is the case with some other prescription drugs, you might expect that the larger the dose, the larger the cost. Example: A 100mg tablet theoretically should cost twice as much as a 50mg tablet. For this particular class of drugs, the SSRIs, this is not the case. All three strengths of the drug cost the pharmacy approximately the same (within ten to twenty dollars per one hundred tablets) no matter what the strength. Therefore, prices for the 25mg, 50mg, and 100mg tablets may be somewhat similar.

Drug and Strength	Quantity	Retail Price
Zoloft 25mg	30 tablets	$60.29–$94.98
Zoloft 50mg	30 tablets	$61.69–$96.49
Zoloft 100mg	30 tablets	$66.19–$97.79

SIDE EFFECTS

The side effects listed below were discovered during well-controlled clinical studies conducted before the FDA approved the drug for public use. Researchers believe the occurrence of these side effects under the drug's normal everyday use in real world settings to be very similar. Side effects are listed in decreasing order based on the percentage of patients experiencing certain side effects. The percentages listed below are averages based on several different clinical tests and are believed to be reliable.

Side Effect	Percentage Experiencing
Nausea/upset stomach	26%–30%
Headache	20%–30%
Diarrhea	18%–24%
Insomnia	16%–28%

Side Effect	Percentage Experiencing
Difficulty in ejaculating	16%–17%
Dry mouth	14%–16%
Drowsiness	13%–15%
Dizziness	12%–17%
Fatigue	11%–14%
Decreased sex drive	11%
Tremors	8%–11%
Nervousness	8%
Increased sweating	6%–8%
Constipation	6%–8%
Agitation	6%
Impotence	5%
Pharyngitis	4%
Gas	4%
Abnormal vision	4%
Decreased appetite	3%–11%
Pounding heartbeat	3%–4%
Vomiting	3%–4%
Depersonalization	3%
General pain	3%
Increased appetite	3%
Numbness	3%
Chest pain	3%
Increased weight	3%
Taste changes	3%
Increased urination	2%
Paranoid feelings	2%
Increased yawning	2%
Sexual dysfunction in females	2%
Decreased function of the senses	2%
Hot flashes	2%
Fever	2%
Back pain	2%
Extreme muscle tension	1%–2%
Twitching	1%

The side effects listed above were reported by patients and, for the most part, were mild to moderate in severity. However, some side effects were severe enough for the patients taking Zoloft to discontinue treatment. In fact, 15 percent of the 2,710 patients taking Zoloft during clinical testing did stop taking the drug due to side effects. These side effects that caused patients to stop taking the drug included agitation, difficulty in ejaculating, insomnia, drowsiness, dizziness, headache, tremor, loss of appetite, nausea, diarrhea, and fatigue.

Researchers also discovered other side effects during clinical testing. These side effects occurred in a very small number of patients who had taken Zoloft. Some of these side effects are very serious; it's important to remember, however, that only a very small number of patients taking Zoloft even experienced these side effects. This should not discourage patients in any way from taking the drug Zoloft. Many prescription drugs have most of these same side effects that occur infrequently or rarely with their use.

The side effects that occurred in about 1 percent of the patients taking Zoloft include confusion, stomach pain, rash, runny nose, muscle pain, increased thirst, ringing in the ears, impaired concentration, and menstrual disorders.

The following list of side effects occurred infrequently (0.1 percent to 1 percent) in patients taking Zoloft. (Note: 1 percent = 1 in every 100 patients and 0.1 percent = 1 in every 1,000 patients.)

flushed skin	high blood pressure
increased salivation	low blood pressure
cold clammy skin	swelling
dizziness when getting up from sitting or lying position	fast heartbeat
	severe dizziness
	bloody nose

abnormal coordination
movement disorders
migraines
vertigo
acne
hair loss
itching
red raised-bumpy
   skin rash
dry skin
eructation
tiredness
muscle stiffness
weight loss
swollen lymph nodes
muscle pain
muscle cramps
muscle weakness
abnormal dreams
aggressive reactions
amnesia

lack of emotion
delusion
depression
emotional instability
euphoria
hallucinations
paranoid reaction
suicide attempt
teeth-grinding
abnormal thinking
abnormal menstrual periods
abnormal vaginal bleeding
coughing
trouble breathing
double vision
earache
eye pain
swelling of the face
increased urination
inflammation and redness of
   the eye

The following list of side effects occurred very rarely
(0.001 percent to 0.1 percent or less) in patients taking
Zoloft. (Note: 0.1 percent = 1 in every 1,000 patients
and 0.001 percent = 1 in every 100,000 patients.)

pale skin
heart attack
varicose veins
coma
convulsions
difficulty speaking
abnormal hair texture
increased sensitivity of the
   skin to sunburn

rash around hair follicles
skin discolorations
abnormal skin odor
enlarged breasts in men
diverticulitis
bowel troubles
gum swelling
hemorrhoids
hiccups

peptic ulcer
stomach ulcers
tongue sores
tongue swelling
enlarged stomach
bad breath
ear infections
anemia
eye hemorrhage
hysteria
withdrawal syndrome
dehydration
high cholesterol
low blood sugar

hernia
breast enlargement in
   females
female breast pain
thinning of the vaginal
   lining
hyperventilation
sinus infections
vision disturbances
increased sensitivity of the
   eyes to sunlight
kidney pain
difficulty in urinating

These side effects are presented for information purposes only, not to scare individuals currently taking Zoloft or to prevent them from taking it in the future. My hope is to increase the patient's awareness, and to report that in some rare instances the drug has caused serious side effects. Zoloft and the SSRIs in general are some of the safest drugs on the market used to treat depression and OCD. However, you should discuss any abnormal side effects that you experience while taking Zoloft with your physician and pharmacist.

DRUG INTERACTIONS

Compared with other drugs used to treat depression and OCD, Zoloft and the SSRIs in general have fewer drug interactions. A drug interaction occurs when two drugs taken together produce an unwanted side effect or adverse effect, or when they affect how one drug or the other works in the body that is different from its intended use. The drug interactions listed below are the most clinically significant and potentially the most serious.

1. Zoloft should never be taken with Eldepryl, Furoxone, Matulane, Nardil, or Parnate. This can cause a very serious and potentially life-threatening condition called serotonin syndrome. Symptoms of this condition can include mental status changes, confusion, restlessness, shivering, tremor, diarrhea, agitation, severe convulsions, and very high blood pressure. If serotonin syndrome is recognized early enough, the patient usually recovers quickly once the drugs are discontinued. However, there have been deaths associated with this lethal combination. Physicians administer no actual treatment for serotonin syndrome, except for supportive care of body functions (maintaining adequate blood pressure, heart function, breathing, etc.).

   Patients taking Zoloft should not take Eldepryl, Furoxone, Matulane, Nardil, or Parnate until at least two weeks after discontinuing treatment with Zoloft. Conversely, patients who have taken these drugs should not be started on Zoloft until at least two weeks after discontinuing MAO inhibitors.

2. Zoloft may increase the blood levels of Coumadin. This may lead to increased bleeding, especially when Zoloft is first started or recently discontinued, in patients taking Coumadin. This potential interaction can be very serious. Your physician may need to adjust your Coumadin dosage. Once the dosage of Coumadin is stabilized, Coumadin and Zoloft can be taken safely together.

3. The amino acid tryptophan, contained in some vitamin supplements, should not be taken in large amounts with Zoloft. Tryptophan is one of the chemicals that serotonin is made from in the body. SSRIs like Zoloft increase the amount of serotonin

available in the body. If an excessive amount of tryptophan is taken, the body may produce more serotonin than normal. This overproduction along with Zoloft's effect on serotonin can result in excessive levels of serotonin. This may cause agitation, restlessness, insomnia, anxiety, and stomach problems like nausea, vomiting, and diarrhea. Therefore, vitamin supplements with large amounts of tryptophan should be avoided.

Other potential drug interactions are also worth mentioning. These interactions do not occur as frequently as the others listed above and are not nearly as serious.

1. Zoloft may increase the drowsiness or sleepiness caused by alcohol, nerve medications, pain killers, muscle relaxers, antihistamines, allergy medications, cold medications, and cough syrups. This may be dangerous when driving, operating heavy machinery, or during any other task were mental alertness is required. This is not to say patients cannot take Zoloft and these other drugs together, but they need to be aware that drowsiness may increase.

2. Zoloft may increase the blood levels of Valium, which may produce significantly more drowsiness and other unwanted side effects. The doctor may need to adjust the Valium dosage when it is taken with Zoloft.

3. Zoloft may increase the blood levels of Orinase. This may lead to low blood sugar in some individuals. Individuals taking Zoloft and Orinase together should monitor their blood glucose levels carefully.

4. Tagamet may increase the blood levels of Zoloft. Individuals taking Tagamet and Zoloft together should be cautious of this potential interaction.

5. Zoloft may alter the blood levels of lithium, which may lead to toxic effects. Blood levels of lithium should be measured and monitored.

6. Zoloft may increase the blood levels of other antidepressants such as Anafranil, Asendin, Elavil, Ludiomil, Norpramin, Pamelor, Sinequan, Surmontil, Tofranil, and Vivactil. This interaction may increase the incidence of side effects associated with taking these antidepressants.

7. Recently, there have been rare reports of Zoloft causing weakness, muscle reflex problems, and coordination problems when taken with Imitrex. Individuals should be aware of this potential drug interaction and use caution when taking Zoloft and Imitrex together.

Researchers also studied the interaction of Zoloft with other drugs, including Tenormin, Lanoxin, and Tegretol for potential drug interactions. These tests found no interactions between these drugs and Zoloft.

FOOD INTERACTIONS

Food does affect the blood levels of the drug. The maximum concentration of drug in the bloodstream may increase by as much as 25 percent if the drug is taken with food, but this increase is not of great concern. Therefore, Zoloft may be taken with or without food or milk. Those who experience mild nausea when taking the drug on an empty stomach may choose to take it with food or milk.

DEALING WITH OVERDOSES

It is possible to overdose on Zoloft when taking large quantities alone or with other drugs and/or alcohol. The symptoms of an overdose include tiredness, nausea, vomiting, fast heartbeat, ECG changes, anxiety, and dilated pupils. There have been no reported deaths when Zoloft was taken alone in an overdose of 500mg to 6000mg. Therefore, the risk of death from an overdose of Zoloft alone is extremely low. Four deaths, however, have been associated with an overdose of Zoloft when combined with another drug and/or alcohol. If you suspect that you or someone else has taken an overdose of Zoloft, contact your nearest poison control center immediately.

ALLERGIES

Individuals who have a past history of being allergic to Zoloft should not take the drug. Individuals allergic to other similar drugs in the same class, such as Prozac, Paxil, or Luvox, should alert their doctor of this and use caution when taking Zoloft. Most of the patients who experienced an allergic reaction reported only itching and a skin rash. However, some patients also reported fever, swollen glands, muscle pain, swelling, and/or trouble breathing. These symptoms disappeared in most patients once they stopped taking the drug or were treated with antihistamines and/or steroids. If a rash, itching, swelling, fever, or swollen glands occurs while taking the drug, contact your doctor. If chest pain, difficulty in breathing, or the other symptoms listed above become worse, seek emergency medical treatment as quickly as possible.

CANCER-CAUSING POTENTIAL

There is no evidence that Zoloft has the potential to cause cancer at this time, even at very high doses. Extensive testing in laboratory mice found no evidence of cancer-causing potential of Zoloft. Cancer-causing studies in mice usually are good predictors of the likely effects in humans regarding cancer-causing potential.

Limited clinical testing in human lymphocytes also showed no evidence of the drug causing cancer.

EFFECT ON SEXUAL FUNCTION

There is some evidence that Zoloft has an effect on some sexual functions, including the ability to have an orgasm, the ability to maintain an erection, the ability to ejaculate, and sexual desire in general. In clinical testing, 16 percent to 17 percent of men taking the drug experienced some form of difficulty in ejaculating, 11 percent of the men and women combined experienced a decrease in sexual desire, 5 percent of men noted impotence problems, and 2 percent of the women experienced some other form of sexual dysfunction, possibly inability to have an orgasm. Some men during clinical testing felt the problem of difficulty in ejaculating during sex was severe enough for them to stop taking the drug. Individuals taking Zoloft should be aware of these potential problems in sexual functioning and report them to their doctor if they become extremely bothersome.

EFFECT ON FERTILITY

There is no evidence that Zoloft will cause fertility problems in either men or women. A decrease in fertility was seen, however, in one of two studies conducted on rats. Rats in these studies received a dose of Zoloft twenty times greater than a human dose. It is important to realize that there are risks associated with taking any drug if a woman believes she is pregnant. If a woman suspects she is pregnant, she should obtain a pregnancy test immediately and discuss with her physician whether she should continue taking Zoloft or not. For a complete discussion on the effects of the drug during pregnancy, see the next section.

SAFETY OF USE DURING PREGNANCY

Zoloft is classified under the Food and Drug Administration's Pregnancy Classification as Category C. Category C means that animal studies have shown Zoloft to have adverse effect on an animal fetus. There are, however, no adequate studies in humans, but the benefits of taking the drug during pregnancy must truly outweigh the risks based on the results of animal testing. The drug was recently reclassified to the more stringent Category C from Category B after further animal studies showed abnormal effects of the drug on the fetus. Animal studies using as much as four times the maximum daily dose of Zoloft showed some harm to the unborn fetus.

When Zoloft was given to rats in the third trimester of pregnancy, an increase in the number of stillborn young, a decrease in total birth weight, and an increase in the number young dying in the first four days after birth were all observed. We lack extensive studies on the effect of Zoloft on the human fetus. If you suspect that you are pregnant, contact your doctor immediately. The manufacturer strongly recommends that Zoloft be used during pregnancy only if the benefits of taking the drug significantly outweigh the risks of potential harm to the fetus.

SAFETY OF USE WHEN BREAST-FEEDING

It is not known if Zoloft is excreted in breast milk. Because many drugs are excreted in breast milk, women taking Zoloft should use extreme caution when breast-feeding.

EXCRETION FROM THE BODY

Zoloft is primarily metabolized by the liver and is removed from the body by the kidneys and the feces through the bowels. This process is very slow, which results in the drug staying in the body for quite some time. In fact, the drug will stay in the body for about twenty-four hours after taking a single dose and one to three days after several days of therapy with Zoloft. Zoloft is metabolized by the liver into the chemical N-desmethylsertraline. This compound only provides about one-eighth of the activity of Zoloft in treating depression and OCD. The metabolite N-desmethylsertraline is not considered an active drug and provides little therapeutic effect in treating depression and OCD. N-desmethylsertraline will stay in the body anywhere from three to five days depending on how long the patient has been taking Zoloft. Patients who have been taking the drug for several weeks should not expect the body to be free of the drug until about one week after the last dose was taken.

WHAT TO KNOW BEFORE YOU USE THIS DRUG

Because the drug is metabolized by the liver, patients with liver disease, hepatitis, or cirrhosis may require lower doses. Patients with kidney disease may require lower doses as well. Also, patients who suffer from seizure disorders or epilepsy may want to inform their doctor of this condition before taking Zoloft. The weight loss that occurs rarely when taking Zoloft should be considered carefully. In some patients, this side effect may be undesirable.

Zoloft is not considered a "quick fix" in treating depression or OCD. The drug may require several weeks of therapy before a significant improvement is seen. Therefore, patients should not become discouraged if they do not see immediate improvement and quit taking the drug. The drug should be taken for at least four to six weeks before the patient and his or her physician decide the drug is not working and that some other medication should be used.

PROPER USE OF THE DRUG

Zoloft should be taken every day in order to receive its maximum benefits. Patients should follow the physician's dosing schedule as closely as possible. Do not take more or less of the drug than is prescribed. Some patients may try to increase the dose on their own if they feel the drug is not effective at the prescribed dose. This may increase the risk of unwanted side effects and other adverse events. Other patients may try to decrease their dose on their own if they experience some unwanted side effects. This may result in too low of a dose being taken. Patients who experience any unwanted side effects or feel that the current dose may be too low should discuss this with their physician or pharmacist before adjusting the amount of medication taken.

If a patient forgets to take his or her daily dose and remembers within two to four hours of when the dose was to be taken, the patient should take the drug as soon as he or she remembers. If the patient forgets to take the daily dose and remembers more than four hours after the medication time, he or she should skip the missed dose and continue on the normal dosing schedule the next day or take the next scheduled dose on time. Patients should not double the dose.

IMPORTANT PATIENT INFORMATION

Individuals taking Zoloft should make regular visits to their physician to check and discuss the progress of their condition. At that time, they should report any side effects or other adverse effects to their physician. If a skin rash, itching, or hives occur after taking the drug, stop taking the drug and contact your physician as soon as possible. These may be the symptoms of an allergic reaction to the drug. If these symptoms are accompanied by tightness in the chest or trouble breathing, seek medical attention immediately.

Zoloft may cause some drowsiness and tiredness, especially at first. The degree of drowsiness caused by Zoloft is significantly less severe than that caused by pain killers, sleeping pills, and other nerve medications. Use caution when driving, operating heavy machinery or equipment, or doing jobs that require a great deal of mental alertness. The degree of drowsiness caused by the drug varies from patient to patient.

It is also important to know that alcohol, nerve medications, pain killers, muscle relaxers, antihistamines, allergy and cold medications, cough syrups, and other drugs known to cause drowsiness may significantly increase the drowsiness caused by Zoloft. Therefore, use extreme caution when taking Zoloft with these drugs. The drug may also cause some limited dizziness or lightheadedness, especially when getting up suddenly from lying or sitting positions.

Some patients taking Zoloft may experience a dry mouth for a short period of time. This side effect is similar in severity to the dry mouth caused by some antihistamines and can be alleviated by chewing sugarless gum or candy. If the dry mouth continues for more than two weeks, patients should contact their physician.

If you experience stomach upset or mild nausea after taking Zoloft, you may take the drug with food or milk to reduce this irritating side effect. If the nausea or stomach upset is severe, continues every time the drug is taken for several days, or vomiting occurs, contact your physician or pharmacist.

Many times Zoloft is prescribed to be taken in the

morning. It does not have to be taken on an empty stomach. Food and milk do not significantly affect the action of the drug in the body or its absorption in the stomach. Therefore, the drug may be taken with breakfast or a morning snack.

STORAGE OF THE DRUG

Zoloft, as with any medications, should be kept out of the reach of children. The drug should be stored away from direct light and heat. Never store any medication in a bathroom medicine cabinet. Heat, moisture, and steam from the shower, bathtub, and sink may cause medications to become ineffective. Medications should also not be stored near the kitchen sink or in any other damp place for the same reason. Ideally, your prescription medications should be stored in a tight, light-resistant (amber or brown) prescription bottle between 59 and 86 degrees and at no more than 104 degrees. Medications are best stored in the original bottles in which they were dispensed. Remember, the temperatures in a hot car or truck can exceed 105 degrees very easily. Therefore, medications should never be left in a hot car or truck for more than thirty to sixty minutes.

FURTHER INFORMATION

Individuals who would like further information on Zoloft should first contact their pharmacist and then their physician. Another source of in-depth information is your local hospital. Many large hospitals, especially those associated with universities, have drug information centers. When calling the hospital, ask for the pharmacy department or drug information center of the hospital. Finally, individuals can contact the company who manufactures and markets the drug directly. Zoloft is manufactured by

Pfizer Inc. and marketed by Roerig, a marketing subsidiary of Pfizer Inc. Their address is: Roerig Division, Pfizer Inc., ATT: Medical Information, 235 East 42nd Street, New York, NY 10017. The phone number is (800) 438-1985.

SEVEN

❧

The Differences Between Prozac, Paxil, Zoloft, and Luvox

Many physicians and researchers will argue that there are no significant differences between Prozac, Paxil, Zoloft, and Luvox. These health professionals feel that one drug is just as good as the other. If this is truly the case, how does a physician decide which one of the four drugs they should prescribe? Many times their decision is based on past experience. They rely on what their patients tell them about how the drug(s) are affecting their lives. These experiences help guide the physician toward one drug or another depending on the characteristics and symptoms of each individual patient.

One reason these drugs are thought to be so similar is the relatively short time they have been used. Prozac came on the market in 1988. It wasn't until about 1995 that the other three entered the market. Therefore, the four SSRIs have been compared with one another for only the last three to four years. Through widespread use of these drugs, more distinct differences between the four SSRIs will emerge. Currently, some physicians feel that there are some differences between the four drugs. As we gain more experience and conduct more research, many more physicians will begin to see some of the differences between them.

From what we already know, there is no set formula to predetermine which of the four SSRIs will work best in each individual patient. The best example to illustrate this point is to look at patients with arthritis. No fewer than twenty drugs on the market are used to treat the pain associated with arthritis. These drugs are called anti-inflammatory drugs. In choosing the right drug, physicians rely on past experience in other patients with arthritis, but each patient is distinctly different. In one patient, the drug Lodine works wonderfully. But for some unknown reason, Lodine doesn't work as well in another patient. Therefore, the physician may try Daypro. If that doesn't work, the physician will keep trying other anti-inflammatory drugs until he or she finds the one that works.

Initial therapy with the SSRIs can be the same way. One patient may see tremendous results with Prozac. Another patient may see hardly any improvement at all with Prozac but better results with Zoloft. The point is that each individual patient is different. Just because one SSRI doesn't produce the desired effect does not mean another one will not. Dr. Williams says, "It's kind of trial and error with many patients. Sometimes I'll start a patient on Prozac and just won't see much improvement. Then I'll try Paxil and see a tremendous response. Everyone's body reacts differently to different drugs. Also, if I know one particular drug worked in one blood relative, I might try that drug first."

I recently had a patient who reacted differently with three different SSRIs. The patient was first prescribed Zoloft for major depression. After several weeks at a "middle of the spectrum" dose, the patient was not seeing an improvement. The physician then raised the dose. Again, after several weeks, the patient was not seeing any improvement. The patient did not have any bothersome side effects while taking Zoloft even at the higher dose.

The physician then switched the patient to Prozac. After a few weeks, the patient began to feel a lot better. Prozac seemed like a wonder drug compared to Zoloft. The patient was still feeling pretty good after one year of continuously taking Prozac. The patient's physician felt he could be doing even better on a little higher dose. The dose was increased and the patient still felt about the same.

Then, perhaps because the patient was experiencing anxiety, his physician switched him to a low dose of Paxil. It took two dosage increases before the patient starting feeling as well as he did when he was taking Prozac. After the last dosage increase, the patient saw his blood sugar shoot way up. I suggested to the patient that he should talk to his physician about switching him back to Prozac. As you can see, the same patient had different effects with three different SSRIs.

The bottom line is there are some distinct differences between Prozac, Paxil, Zoloft, and Luvox. Past research and thousands of patient experiences have already given us some insight into these differences. As physicians and researchers become more familiar with these drugs, this knowledge base is expected to grow. This chapter provides insight into some of the differences between the four SSRIs.

APPROVED USES

One of the differences between the four SSRIs is what diseases they are approved to treat. Prozac, Paxil, and Zoloft are all approved to treat depression. Luvox is the only drug of the four without formal approval to treat depression. However, Luvox is approved to treat depression throughout most of Europe and Canada. Expect approval of Luvox to treat depression in the near future.

All four drugs are approved to treat obsessive-compulsive disorder (OCD) in adults. Luvox, however, is the only one approved to treat OCD in children ages eight to seventeen. This does not mean the other three are not used in children with OCD, but Luvox is the only one with formal approval.

Zoloft and Paxil are also approved to treat panic disorder. This a relatively new indication or use for the SSRIs. Prozac, on the other hand, is approved to treat bulimia nervosa and may eventually be approved to treat anorexia nervosa.

As you can see, these drugs are slowly gaining approval for use in conditions other than depression and OCD. As more research is conducted, expect to see even broader use of these drugs in other types of mental illnesses.

USUAL DOSE

This is a very hard comparison to make. It's like comparing apples and oranges. For example, patients usually take 20mg to 40mg of Prozac once daily 50mg to 100mg of Zoloft once daily for depression. Patients can't assume that because they are taking twice as much Zoloft they will experience more side effects. The dose of Prozac is lower because the drug is more potent. Patients taking 20mg of Prozac are probably just as likely to experience side effects as those taking 50mg of Zoloft. You really cannot compare the four drugs on a milligram (mg) by milligram basis.

I've seen patients do very well on low doses of one SSRI but experience no effects from high doses of another. I've also seen some patients achieve tremendous results on 20mg a day of Prozac and others experience no relief on 60mg of Prozac a day. Everyone's body chemistry is different.

There is, however, one small difference between the four. Prozac, Paxil, and Zoloft are usually given only once daily no matter how high the dose. Higher doses of Prozac may be split into two equal doses to be given in the morning and at noon. Luvox, however, should be given twice daily, in the morning and at bedtime, if the total dose to be taken is higher that 100mg. This may present problems with patients being willing or able to keep their medication schedule.

Patients who only have to take a drug once daily are more likely to take their medication regularly and not miss doses, as compared to those who must take a drug two or more times per day. Patients taking higher doses of Luvox must remember to take their medication twice daily instead of once, and therefore are not as likely to be compliant.

Prozac also has one other slight advantage over the other three SSRIs: It is available as a liquid. This may be important for patients who have trouble swallowing capsules and tablets, those patients with feeding tubes, and for children. There is one catch: Prozac liquid is priced significantly higher than the tablet and capsule formulations of the others when compared on a dose-by-dose basis. Based on personal experience, Dr. Williams believes that Zoloft and Luvox are harder to dose than Prozac and Paxil. Therefore, he is more likely to pre-scribe Prozac or Paxil first.

CLINICAL EFFECTIVENESS

A limited amount of sound research has been conducted comparing the effectiveness of the four SSRI drugs. The conclusion has been the same in almost every study. There is no evidence that one drug is superior to another.

However, some patients may see more effect from one of the SSRIs over another. This is due to the fact that everyone's body chemistry and disease state is different. Sometimes physicians will try two or three of the SSRIs until finding the right one for each individual patient. There are a few other subtle differences worth mentioning regarding effectiveness.

All four drugs usually require one to four weeks before patients see noticeable benefits. Some patients report experiencing benefits almost immediately, but most report relief of symptoms in about one to four weeks, no matter which drug is used. Some evidence, however, suggests that Paxil may start working sooner than the other three. Dr. Williams, however, does not believe that this is true. Other information suggests that when Paxil is taken with the drug Visken, the onset of action is even quicker. Most of this evidence is purely anecdotal and more research is definitely needed.

Another slight difference is the length of time these drugs stay in the body. Prozac stays in the body a significantly longer period of time that the other three. This may be important if a patient is experiencing unwanted side effects from Prozac because side effects may take longer to resolve.

Another difference is that the chemical metabolite of Prozac is also an active ingredient. The active metabolite of Prozac, norfluoxetine, has some activity in treating depression, OCD, and other conditions. This active metabolite may stay in the body for four to fourteen days. If a patient has been taking Prozac regularly, it make take as long as two weeks before all of the drug and its metabolite are completely gone from the body.

Zoloft also has an active metabolite, but its metabolite is a lot less effective and active than Prozac's. Zoloft's active metabolite will stay in the body for about three to five days. Paxil and Luvox do not have an active metabolite. The bottom line is that Prozac stays in the body the longest of the four. This may mean that adverse side effects may take longer to resolve once Prozac is stopped than with the other three SSRIs.

I asked Dr. Williams how long it takes before the SSRIs start to work and if the length of time is the same for all patients. He said, "The fastest onset of effect I've ever seen was one week. Many times it takes between two to four weeks. If the patient does not notice a difference after six weeks, the physician should think about trying another drug. Paxil has been said to work faster, but that is not the case. Paxil will decrease some of the nervousness and insomnia that accompany depression, so this in and of itself will make patients feel better. But it still takes one to four weeks before true improvement in their depression will occur."

USE IN THE ELDERLY

All four drugs have been shown to be effective when used by elderly patients. There has not been any substantial research published regarding the superiority of one the SSRIs over the other in the elderly. At this point, all four are considered essentially equal in effectiveness when used in the elderly.

However, one difference is worth mentioning. Studies have shown that Paxil and Luvox produce significantly higher blood levels in elderly patients as compared to younger patients. This may require more careful monitoring or possibly lower doses in the elderly of these two drugs. Currently with Prozac and Zoloft, no reduction in dose is needed. However, other medical problems or diseases may require lower doses of any of the four SSRIs in elderly patients. I have seen in my practice that some elderly individuals tend to be more sensitive to some medications. Therefore, I think it's wise to begin someone who is elderly on a lower dose and then gradually increase the dose if necessary.

USE IN CHILDREN

Luvox is currently the only one of the four SSRIs approved to be used in children. Luvox is approved to treat OCD in children ages eight to seventeen. But this is not to say that doctors are not prescribing the others for children. Research has shown that hundreds of thousands of children are being given these drugs for a variety of conditions. This is an extremely large and expanding potential market for these drugs. Where the potential for money is at stake, research usually follows. Currently, there is little functional research regarding the effectiveness of the SSRIs in children, but expect to see a great deal of it in the near future. For a discussion on what is known currently, refer to Chapter 8.

PRICES

The future pricing of these drugs is very hard to predict. In the market for prescription drugs, the cost to manufacture the product has little to do with how it is priced. Competitive factors, size of the product's market share, generic availability, new uses and indication, and financial performance of the company making the drug contribute more to pricing than the cost of raw materials used to make the drug.

Currently, the four drugs are about the same price. However, Paxil and Luvox seem to be slightly less expensive. This is probably because they were the last two on the market. In the future, I would expect all four drugs to continue to be priced very similarly.

SIDE EFFECTS

This is one of the areas where we tend to see the most difference between the four drugs. Based on discussions with patients, physicians, and research conducted by the manufacturers of the drugs, we have made many observations. Note that these are only observations and should be interpreted carefully. More research needs to be conducted comparing the side effects of all four SSRIs.

It seems that Zoloft and Luvox tend to cause more GI problems, mostly stomach upset, nausea, and diarrhea. Zoloft, Paxil, and Prozac appear to decrease appetite and food intake while Luvox does not. Physicians also report that Paxil tends to cause more drowsiness than the other three. Many physicians like the drowsiness produced because it seems to calm the nervousness that accompanies depression and OCD in many patients taking it. Paxil also appears to cause dry mouth and constipation more often. Finally, most cases of withdrawal syndrome usually involve Paxil.

These are only a few examples of the differences in side effects between the four SSRIs. Rather than discuss each individual side effect separately, I have compiled a convenient table listing all of the prominent side effects of all four drugs. (See page 147). Percentages are given only if the side effects were experienced by 1 percent or more of patients taking the drug in clinical trials. A (−) means less than 1 percent of the patients taking the drug in clinical trials experienced that particular side effect.

The most problematic side effects of the SSRIs are sexual: decreased sex drive, impotence, difficulty in having an orgasm, and problems ejaculating. The incidence of these side effects is about the same across all four SSRIs. Dr. Williams says, ''Hardly any of patients ever discuss these side effects with me. I know some patients experience them, but I think they are too embarrassed to talk about it. Only if I specifically ask them about these side effects will they open up. Patients need to be open with their doctor, even if the side effects are embarrassing to discuss. We cannot help them if we don't know what they are feeling and experiencing.''

**ALPHABETICAL LISTING OF SIDE EFFECTS FOR
LUVOX, PAXIL, PROZAC, AND ZOLOFT**

Side Effect	Luvox	Paxil	Prozac	Zoloft
Abnormal dreams	—	4%	—	—
Abnormal ejaculating	8%	—	—	—
Abnormal vision	—	4%	3%	4%
Agitation	2%	—	—	6%
Amnesia	—	2%	—	—
Anxiety	—	—	13%	—
Back pain	—	—	—	2%
Blurred vision	3%	4%	—	—
Chest pain	—	—	—	3%
Chills	2%	—	—	—
Confusion	—	1%	—	—
Constipation	10%	14–16%	—	6–8%
Decreased appetite	—	6–9%	—	3–11%
Decreased function of the senses	—	—	—	2%
Decreased sex drive	2%	3–7%	4%	11%
Depersonalization	—	—	—	3%
Depression	2%	—	—	—
Diarrhea	11%	10–12%	12%	18–24%

Side Effect	Luvox	Paxil	Prozac	Zoloft
Difficulty ejaculating	—	13–23%	—	16–17%
Difficulty swallowing	2%	—	—	—
Difficulty urinating	—	3%	—	—
Dizziness	11%	12–13%	10%	12–17%
Drowsiness	22%	23–24%	13%	13–15%
Drugged feeling	—	2%	—	—
Dry mouth	14%	18%	10%	14–16%
Extreme muscle tension	—	—	—	1–2%
Fatigue	—	—	—	11–14%
Feeling of a lump in the throat	—	2%	—	—
Fever	—	—	2%	2%
Flulike symptoms	3%	—	5%	—
Flushed feeling	3%	—	—	—
Gas	4%	4%	3%	4%
General pain	—	—	—	3%
Headache	22%	18%	21%	20–30%
Hot flashes	—	—	—	2%
Impotence	2%	8%	—	5%
Increased appetite	—	4%	—	3%
Increased sweating	7%	9–11%	8%	6–8%
Increased urination	3%	3%	—	2%
Increased yawning	2%	4%	3%	2%
Indigestion	—	—	8%	—
Insomnia	21%	13–24%	20%	16–28%

Side Effect	Luvox	Paxil	Prozac	Zoloft
Itching	—	—	3%	—
Loss of appetite	6%	—	11%	—
Low blood pressure	—	—	3%	—
Muscle disease	—	2%	—	—
Muscle numbness	—	1%	—	—
Muscle pain	—	1%	—	—
Muscle tightness	2%	—	—	—
Nausea/upset stomach	40%	23–26%	23%	26–30%
Nervousness	12%	5–9%	13%	8%
Numbness	—	4%	—	3%
Paranoid feelings	—	—	—	2%
Pharyngitis	—	—	5%	4%
Pounding heartbeat	3%	2–3%	2%	3–4%
Rash	—	2–3%	4%	—
Sexual dysfunction in females	—	2–3%	—	2%
Sexual dysfunction in males	—	10%	—	—
Taste changes	3%	2%	—	3%
Toothache, cavities, or abscess	3%	—	—	—
Tremors	5%	8–11%	10%	8–11%
Trouble breathing	2%	—	—	—
Trouble concentrating	—	3%	—	—

Side Effect	Luvox	Paxil	Prozac	Zoloft
Trouble having an orgasm	2%	—	—	—
Twitching	—	—	—	1%
Upper respiratory infection	9%	—	—	—
Urinary retention	1%	—	—	—
Vomiting	5%	—	3%	3–4%
Weakness/loss of strength	14%	15–22%	12%	—
Weight increase	—	—	—	3%
Weight loss	—	—	2%	—

DRUG INTERACTIONS

For the most part the four SSRI drugs have about the same drug interactions. However, a few particular drug interactions occur only with certain SSRIs. Luvox seems to have more potentially serious drug interactions than the other three. Luvox should never be taken with Propulsid, Seldane, Seldane-D, or Hismanal. This interaction may cause serious irregular heartbeats that may be fatal. Luvox may also increase the blood levels of Clozaril, Tegretol, Inderal, Lopressor, methadone, Valium, Xanax, Halcion, Versed, and theophylline drugs. There have also been reports of slow heart rate in patients taking Luvox and Cardizem, Cardizem SR, Cardizem CD, Dilacor XR, or Tigzac. Other differences seen between the four SSRIs and the drugs they may interact with are as follows:

1. Zoloft may increase the blood levels of Valium and Orinase.

2. Tagamet may increase the blood levels of Zoloft and Paxil.
3. Paxil may increase the blood levels of Kemadrin and theophylline drugs.
4. Dilantin and phenobarbital may decrease the blood levels of Paxil.
5. Prozac may increase the blood levels of Dilantin.
6. Prozac may increase the amount and severity of side effects from Compazine, Etrafon, Haldol, Loxitane, Mellaril, Moban, Navane, Orap, Prolixin, Serentil, Stelazine, Thorazine, and Trilafon.

USE WITH FOOD

Food and milk do not affect the amount or rate of absorption of Prozac, Paxil, or Luvox. These drugs may be taken on a full or empty stomach. If nausea occurs while taking one of these three, the drug should be taken with food (preferably a meal) or a large glass of milk.

Zoloft, however, is different. Food actually helps with the absorption of the Zoloft. In fact, blood levels of Zoloft may increase by as much as 25 percent if the patient takes the drug with food. Research has shown that this increase, however, is not of great concern. Zoloft may be taken with or without food. Zoloft also seems to cause slightly more nausea in patients than the other three SSRIs. Therefore, I recommend that patients taking Zoloft do so with food or milk.

USE IN PREGNANCY

Paxil, Zoloft, and Luvox are classified, based on risk, as Category C. Prozac, on the other hand, is classified as Category B. In this system, A is considered the most safe and D is considered the least safe. Research indicates that Prozac may be somewhat more safe to use in pregnancy than the other three. Prozac has been tested in a few small studies of pregnant women, whereas the other three have not. There is still some risk to the fetus while taking Prozac during pregnancy. Even though Prozac is somewhat safer than the other three SSRIs, pregnant women should still exercise extreme caution.

BREAST-FEEDING

Prozac, Paxil, and Luvox are known to be excreted in the breast milk. These three drugs should never be prescribed for women who are breast-feeding. It is not known whether Zoloft is excreted in the breast milk. But the majority of health care professionals feel that women who are taking Zoloft should not breast-feed.

This chapter has provided a brief summary of some of the differences between Prozac, Paxil, Zoloft, and Luvox. The goal of this chapter was to provide some insight into the differences of the four SSRIs. I hope that this discussion will stimulate communication between patients and their doctor and pharmacist regarding which SSRI may be right for them. This information is in no way a substitute for the advice of your own doctor or pharmacist. Also, patients should never switch drugs on their own or take another person's medication without consulting their doctor or pharmacist.

EIGHT

❧

Children and SSRIs

DEPRESSION AND CHILDREN

Depression is now considered a major problem in children. Failure in school, as well as dropout, are common outcomes for children and teens who are depressed. Recently, we are seeing a decrease in the age when depression first occurs. In fact, many depressed adults may have actually first experienced depression in their teens. At the time, it may have gone undiagnosed. Dr. Williams continues to diagnose depression in younger and younger children, sometimes as young as seven or eight. It's also interesting that depression in teens is more common in females than males. This trend continues into adulthood.

"Treating childhood depression early is very important," says Dr. Williams. "In children as young as six, depression can interfere with the capacity to develop mentally and socially. Their overall development includes building social skills. Depression can greatly hinder this development and produce adverse effects that can last a lifetime," he says.

Depression is one of the most common mental illnesses in children, affecting about 2 percent of children in the United States. Children with immediate family members who have major depression are more likely to suffer from major depression themselves. The concern with this illness in children is that depression is hard to diagnose and often goes untreated. Children, especially younger ones, tend to mask the symptoms of depression more often than adults. There's no doubt that a thirty-year-old adult and an eight-year-old child with depression both experience the symptoms. However, the adult is likely to say, "Hey, there's something wrong with me," and seek treatment. The child is more likely to say, "My parents and teachers are all jerks," not understanding that the problem may be coming from within.

Dr. Williams thinks that many times the symptoms of childhood depression are mistaken for something else. Not all children who are depressed are sad and gloomy. Many times the symptoms of childhood depression may be behavior problems at school or trouble with the law. Often a depressed child becomes withdrawn or stops socializing with friends and other children. Here is a typical example of child suffering from childhood depression.

Missy is a ten-year-old female. Until about a year ago, she was a friendly, well-behaved child who was active in soccer and did very well in school. At that time, she started becoming very irritable and could not seem to get along with her friends or teammates. Recently, she has had a couple of crying spells for no apparent reason. She doesn't even know why she's crying when asked. Now her grades are beginning to drop and she wants to quit the soccer team. Her mother has also noticed that her appetite is not what it used to be, and she has lost five pounds over the past few months. Three times last month her father found her wandering around the house at one o'clock in the morning saying she couldn't get to sleep. Missy is most likely suffering from major depression.

SIGNS AND SYMPTOMS OF DEPRESSION IN CHILDREN

The symptoms of depression usually vary based on the age of the child. The information provided below is designed to help you assess whether your child may or may not be suffering from major depression. This information is not intended to replace a qualified physician's diagnosis of your child's condition. Only a doctor can properly diagnose if your child is suffering from major depression.

EARLY CHILDHOOD (AGES THREE TO FOUR)

The language skills of children in this age group may not be well enough developed for them to express their mood. Physicians are still not in total agreement that depression can occur in children this young. However, many physicians believe than there are some common symptoms seen in children in this age group. These are:

1. abnormal motor behavior (running around wildly for no reason)
2. hyperactivity
3. extreme aggression
4. being opposed to everything they are told to do
5. social withdrawal (always wanting to be by themselves or alone)
6. loss of appetite and trouble sleeping

MIDDLE CHILDHOOD
(AGES FIVE TO EIGHT)

Depression in this age group is usually more recognizable than in the early childhood group. These symptoms may include:

1. low self-esteem
2. extreme feelings of guilt about things
3. extreme and prolonged periods of sadness
4. social withdrawal (always wanting to play alone)
5. accident-proneness
6. always blaming themselves for something
7. underachieving or not doing well in school
8. aggression or being contrary
9. possibly excessive lying and/or stealing

LATE CHILDHOOD
(AGES NINE TO TWELVE)

The symptoms of depression may be hard to identify in this group, just as in the early childhood group, because these children may try to hide their true feelings or what is bothering them. Some symptoms of depression in this age group may be:

1. excessive anxiety
2. feelings of helplessness
3. lack of pleasure in normally enjoyable activities such as a trip to an amusement park
4. a more than usual amount of irritability
5. school problems (behavior and/or poor grades)
6. excessive sadness
7. inability to concentrate
8. possibly the beginning of suicidal thoughts and intentions

ADOLESCENTS (AGES THIRTEEN TO EIGHTEEN)

By the time children reach the age of thirteen, the symptoms of depression are very similar to those of adults. To assess if your teen may be suffering from depression, give them the depression quiz in Chapter 1. Depression in teens can be very serious. Many teens view the world in an all-or-nothing manner, meaning they usually feel that things will never change. Therefore, this age group of depressed patients is at greater risk for suicide. Also, depression in this age group often leads to drug and/or alcohol abuse. If you suspect your teen may be depressed, contact your doctor and have your child professionally evaluated.

OBSESSIVE-COMPULSIVE DISORDER AND CHILDREN

Traditionally, OCD was thought to occur mainly in adults, but this is no longer the case. OCD represents about 1 percent of all pediatric psychiatric referrals and is two to four times more common in young boys than young girls. OCD usually begins during the teen years but can begin during childhood. Symptoms have been reported in children as young as three, but most symptoms don't appear until the early teens, usually around age fourteen to fifteen. For more complete information on OCD, refer to Chapter 1.

In children and teens, the obsessions and compulsions are closely tied together. A teen who has a fear of contamination will mostly likely wash his hands several times during the day or touch certain things only with a tissue. Other teens, however, may describe a complex routine of touching themselves in order to prevent harm to themselves. Some teens may try to block out a particular thought or worry before a compulsive behavior like walking in and out of the same doorway fifteen times.

Some children and teens are considered perfectionists. They want to get everything right. These children do not necessarily have OCD. A child or teen with OCD allows these thoughts of perfection to consume large portions of their day and interfere with their normal daily lives. In this case these thoughts have become obsessional. Other children tend to worry about a lot of things such as a test or starting a new school. Children who worry a lot do not have OCD either, but when these worries occupy most of their thoughts, OCD may be a possibility. I remember one teen with OCD who would carefully think through every single word before she spoke. This teen was always afraid of saying the wrong thing or offending someone. Below is an example of a child with OCD.

Jimmy is thirteen years old. Every day Jimmy walks home from school following the exact same path. As he passes the first stop sign he taps on it thirteen times with his right hand. Further down the street, four large oak trees stand in Mrs. Smith's yard. Before he continues past them, he must walk five circles around each of the four trees. Mrs. Smith told him one day that she was going to have those four trees cut down. He begged her not to do it. He said it was because they were so beautiful, but the real reason was that it would alter his daily routine.

For the next fifty yards, the sidewalk is old and cracked. He takes at least fifteen minutes to walk that fifty yards being very careful not to step on any of the cracks. When he gets home, he opens and closes the mailbox at least a dozen times just to make sure there is no mail. At the dinner table, Jimmy arranges his silverware and dishes in the same exact order for every meal.

He must touch the glass, plate, bowl, and silverware in that order ten times before he eats. If anything upsets any of Jimmy's normal routines, he becomes very irritated and upset. Jimmy has OCD.

SIGNS AND SYMPTOMS OF OCD IN CHILDREN

The information provided below is designed to help you assess whether your child or teen may be suffering from OCD. This information is not intended to replace a qualified physician's diagnosis of your child's condition. Only a doctor can properly diagnose if your child or teen is suffering from OCD.

The symptoms of OCD in children are similar to those in adults. The most common obsessive-compulsive thoughts in children and teens are:

1. Fears of contamination (dirt, feces, and germs)—this may lead to excessive hand-washing, showering, or bathing.
2. Fears of doing something wrong (misbehaving, lying, or stealing)—this may lead the child to constantly ask for the parent's approval or permission for everything, including simple things like getting a drink of water or going to the bathroom.
3. Having to touch objects or perform certain rituals in a specific sequence in order to avoid danger or trouble—this may include touching each piece of silverware in a certain order (fork, spoon, knife) around the plate several times before eating, or brushing teeth several times a day to avoid having to go to the dentist.
4. Having to perform complex bedtime rituals—these rituals usually take several minutes to complete before the child will go to bed. Example: When told

to go to bed, a child first walks through every room in the house and counts to thirty in each room. Then he walks in and out of the bathroom several times for no reason. After this, he walks back to the kitchen and opens the refrigerator several times. Finally, he looks in every closet and under every bed in the house several times to make sure no one is hiding there.

It's true that many children look under the bed for monsters and others don't like to get dirty. These children are most likely not suffering from OCD and parents shouldn't become alarmed. The thing that should help parents distinguish between OCD and these normal behaviors is how excessive they are. If these behaviors occupy more than one hour of your child's day, the child may be suffering from OCD. If your child is exhibiting behaviors in excess and similar to those listed above, he or she may be obsessive-compulsive. Contact your doctor for a thorough and proper assessment and evaluation of your child's behavior(s).

USING SSRIs IN CHILDREN

There has been explosive growth in the prescription of SSRIs for children in recent years. It is estimated that hundreds of thousands of children are taking SSRIs for everything from depression to Attention Deficit Disorder with or without Hyperactivity (ADD or ADDH). In fact, children represent the fastest growing market segment for the SSRIs. The "Prozac Nation," as it's sometimes called, is definitely shifting to a new patient population, children.

Children as young as five, and in some rare cases even three, are beginning to receive SSRIs to treat a whole host of conditions including depression, obsessive-compulsive disorder (OCD), and even Attention Deficit Disorder with or without Hyperactivity (ADD and ADDH). The Food and Drug Administration estimates that as many as three thousand infants under the age of one may have been given Prozac. These children, however, weren't being given Prozac to treat infant depression. Most likely physicians prescribed the drug as a last-chance effort for rare diseases such as neurodevelopmental disorders in which infants do violent harm to themselves. Eli Lilly, the drug's manufacturer, claims this estimate is totally false. There is, however, a real fear by the FDA and many expert physicians that some doctors may prescribe an SSRI just because a baby is cranky.

The debate continues to rage in the medical community over whether Prozac, Paxil, Luvox, and Zoloft are useful in children with depression, OCD, ADD, and ADDH. However, all parties involved do agree on one major point: More research needs to be conducted. According to Dr. Williams, "There is very little research regarding the effectiveness of treating childhood and teen depression and obsessive-compulsive disorder (OCD). Much of what we know about the effectiveness of these drugs has been gained through trial and error. We've seen some dramatic results, but more research definitely needs to be conducted." In fact, Luvox is the only drug formally approved for use in children and it is approved only to treat OCD.

Doctors know that these drugs are extremely effective in adult patients, so in theory they should also work in children. However, the medical community has no definitive answer regarding exactly how these drugs affect children, either positively or negatively. Many new treatment successes are discovered through trial, error, and experience. For many parents and physicians, the potential benefits greatly outweigh the risks. One parent commented, "When your eleven-year-old child says he's so depressed he wants to kill himself . . . You're at the point where you will try about anything." Dr. Williams says, "Children have real problems, too. You would not believe the extent of depression and/or OCD in some children. They really do need treatment and in many cases these drugs have turned their lives around."

Another concern within the medical community is the long-term effects of these drugs. In adults, the side effects from long-term use have not been well studied and in children the risk may be even greater. A child's body is not an exact copy of an adult's. A child is still going through growth and developmental stages that the long-term use of any drug could potentially affect. Scientists don't believe the long-term effects of the SSRIs in children are serious, but until more research is conducted they won't know for sure. After all, Prozac has only been available for about ten years, and Zoloft, Paxil, and Luvox for significantly less time than that. It will be at least another five to ten years before we even have some evidence of what the long-term consequences of these drugs are.

APPROVED USES IN CHILDREN: OBSESSIVE-COMPULSIVE DISORDER

Many times drug manufacturers don't spend the time or money to gain formal approval for the use of their drugs in children. Their reasoning for this is very simple. First of all, when a new drug is being tested, the FDA requires that all testing for initial approval be conducted on adults. This requirement is an ethical one. Unless it's a drug designed specifically for children, the FDA and the medical community feel it's not appropriate to test new drugs on children. (I completely agree.)

However, once a company gains approval for a drug

in adults, they just assume the medical community will consent to its use of the drug in children, but in smaller doses. This is a serious problem. Children are not miniature adults. Their bodies may react differently to a drug than an adult's. This mode of thinking, however, may be changing. As the market for SSRIs for children continues to grow exponentially, expect to see more of the SSRIs approved for use specifically in children.

Currently, Luvox is the only SSRI that is formally approved by the FDA for use in children, specifically for OCD. Luvox is not formally approved for use in children with depression, but it is extensively prescribed. The manufacturer examined the effectiveness in treating OCD in children in a ten-week study. Children between the ages of eight and seventeen were given between 50mg and 200mg per day of Luvox depending on the severity of the disease in each child. Children in this study had moderate to severe OCD. The one shortcoming of the study was the relatively small number of children included. The following table illustrates the results of study participants regarding their symptoms associated with OCD.

IMPROVEMENT IN SYMPTOMS ASSOCIATED WITH OCD

Outcome	No Drug	Luvox
Worse	6%	8%
No change	44%	16%
Minimally improved	22%	37%
Much improved	17%	18%
Very much improved	11%	21%

As you can see, many children did benefit from using Luvox in OCD. The study also looked for differences in effectiveness between boys and girls, and essentially boys and girls reacted the same way when given Luvox to treat their OCD. Another minor factor worth discussing is the degree of effectiveness based on age. One exploratory analysis found that children in the eight-to-eleven age group had a more dramatic improvement in their OCD with Luvox than those ages twelve to seventeen. The Researchers do not completely understand the significance of this finding, and therefore it should not necessarily be interpreted to mean that children ages eight to eleven may respond more favorably than those ages twelve to seventeen.

In the above study, the percentage of children experiencing various side effects were similar to those experienced by adults. There were, however, a few exceptions. Side effects such as abnormal thinking or not thinking clearly, increased cough, missed menstrual periods, some emotional instability, bruising, rash, tics, muscle twitching, manic reaction, infection, bloody nose, stuffy nose, and weight decrease were more commonly seen in children than in adults.

The recommended dosage for children eight to seventeen is initially 25mg at bedtime. Doses of the drug may be increased in increments of 25mg per day every four to seven days. The normal range of doses in children is 50mg to 200mg per day. If the daily dose is more than 50mg, the dose should be equally divided in two. These higher doses should be taken in the morning and at bedtime. If the daily dose cannot be equally divided, the larger of the two doses should be taken at bedtime. The drug is not approved for use in children under the age of eight.

Based on his own experience, Dr. Williams believes that the other SSRIs (Prozac, Paxil, and Zoloft) are just as effective in treating OCD in children as Luvox. Luvox was just the first one of the four to gain formal approval. In fact, Dr. Williams often prefers to use either Prozac,

Paxil, or Zoloft because they may be taken once daily, whereas, Luvox is usually given twice daily. Dr. Williams has seen tremendous results in children and teens with OCD who are treated with SSRIs. Many children and teens see a significant decrease in their obsessions and compulsion when taking an SSRI. Dr. Williams does add, however, that the process of improvement does take time. Parents shouldn't expect these medications to produce dramatic results overnight.

UNAPPROVED USES IN CHILDREN: DEPRESSION AND ATTENTION DEFICIT DISORDER

Before discussing published research reports on the use of SSRIs in children, a couple of important points must be made. First, the amount of research regarding the use of Prozac, Paxil, Zoloft, and Luvox in children is very small. For this reason many physicians are reluctant to prescribe these drugs for children. Also, the few published studies regarding the effectiveness of SSRIs in childhood and adolescent mental conditions have been conducted on small numbers of patients. This raises questions regarding the overall effectiveness of the SSRIs in children.

However, some of these small studies have shown promising results, especially in childhood depression. In addition to these research studies, much of what we know has been learned through simple trial and error by physicians. This old-fashioned technique is important, however, and will continue to remain a vital tool in gaining even more knowledge regarding the safe use of SSRIs in children. The future looks bright for these four drugs and the children and teens who hope to benefit from their use.

TREATING DEPRESSION WITH SSRIs

As just mentioned, much of what we know about treating childhood depression is acquired through physician trial and error. However, a few studies have provided some fairly positive results. In one study of forty teens ages thirteen to eighteen, patients saw a small improvement in symptoms related to depression when taking 40mg to 60mg of Prozac per day.[1] In another study, the records of forty adolescent inpatients with some form of depression who had taken Prozac were examined. Most of the respondents reported a significant decrease in their depression-related symptoms.[2] It must be noted, however, that 75 percent of those children taking Prozac in this study reported some unwanted side effects.

Preliminary results of another study has found that Paxil (given 20mg to 40mg daily) was effective and well tolerated in adolescent patients with depression.[3] In fact, 76 percent of the twenty-five patients ages thirteen to seventeen taking Paxil in this study reported a significant improvement with minimal side effects. In yet another study of thirty-one hospitalized adolescent patients with depression, researchers found that 74 percent of the patients treated with Prozac showed some improvement, and 54 percent of those showed much or very much improvement.[4] These studies show some promising results in treating childhood and adolescent psychiatric disorders with SSRIs. As researchers conduct further studies and gain more experience in their use, the question of effectiveness of SSRIs in children and teens should become more clear.

Dr. Williams has seen some wonderful results in children and teens he has treated with SSRIs for depression. He recalls one little girl who was failing horribly in school. Once her depression was diagnosed and treated with Paxil, her parents saw her grades steadily rise for the rest of the school year. Another child had lost interest in everything that had once give him pleasure, including basketball and baseball. Once his depression was diagnosed and treated with Prozac, he started to regain interest in sports again. He even began talking about trying to get a college scholarship in baseball. His dreams were once again alive and vibrant.

I had a patient who at the age of sixteen would not get out of bed for an entire weekend several times a month. She even let her personal hygiene go to the point that she would wear the same clothes for days at a time and shower only once a week. She felt that her life was meaningless. Once she started taking Zoloft, the turnaround was tremendous. She began going out on the weekends, she got a new haircut, started wearing makeup again, and even found a boyfriend. She once again took pride in her appearance. She had regained some of her self-esteem.

ATTENTION DEFICIT DISORDER WITH OR WITHOUT HYPERACTIVITY (ADD/ADDH)

We lack a great deal of information regarding the success of SSRIs in children with ADD or ADDH, even more so than for depression and OCD, simply because physicians are only beginning to explore the use of these drugs for this condition. Dr. Williams believes the SSRIs may be helpful for some patients, but has only tried them in a few cases because the medical community still doesn't have much information regarding their use in ADD and ADDH.

Dr. Williams has only seen limited improvements in children with ADD and AADH taking SSRIs. SSRIs may calm these children down slightly, but this is probably due to the drowsiness effect of these drugs. It is not clear how much a child's attention span increases while taking SSRIs. At this point, Dr. Williams still prefers to use Ritalin or Dexedrine in his patients with ADD or ADDH.

He has, however, used either Paxil or Prozac in patients with both depression and ADD or ADDH. He has seen an improvement in many of these patients' symptoms. This effect, however, was most likely due to the improvement of the depression. He does feel the drugs are useful in oppositional defiance. Oppositional defiance is defined as opposing and arguing strongly with everything a parent, teacher, or other people in a position of authority tell the child to do. He prescribed Paxil for three patients with oppositional defiance, which resulted in fewer behavioral complaints about the child. At this time, however, the true effectiveness of the SSRIs in ADD and ADDH is still very unclear. Expect to see a lot more research in this area in the near future as physicians look for an alternative to Ritalin and Dexedrine.

WHICH DRUG TO USE IN CHILDREN?

When treating children with depression or OCD, Dr. Williams prefers to use either Prozac or Paxil. Personally, he feels Zoloft is hard to dose in both children and adults, based on his experience with patients. Luvox is usually not one of his first choices because it must be taken twice daily. Also, if a child has some history of agitation, Dr. Williams will usually prescribe Paxil, as Prozac may produce some nervousness or agitation in a small number of children.

Another factor that determines his decision is the types of dosage forms available. Dr. Williams particularly likes to prescribe Prozac in children because it's the only SSRI available in a liquid. Swallowing capsules and tablets can be unpleasant, especially in children younger than twelve. Because they don't like to swallow a tablet or capsule, they don't take their medicine regularly. For these medications to help children, they must be taken regularly every day. Another consideration is whether any immediate family member has taken an SSRI in the past. For example, if a child's mother has taken Zoloft in the past for depression and it worked well, Dr. Williams will most likely try Zoloft on the child first. His experiences have shown him that if one drug works well in one family member it will most likely work as well in another.

Prozac, Paxil, Luvox, and Zoloft will continue to be prescribed more and more for children. The low occurrence of side effects and relative safety of the drugs makes them good choices in children with OCD and depression. However, until more research is conducted, the long-term side effects and effectiveness will still remain a question mark with many health-care professionals.

NINE

❧

Future Uses of Prozac, Paxil, Zoloft, and Luvox

It is not illegal for a physician to prescribe a prescription drug to treat a disease for which it is not formally approved by the Food and Drug Administration (FDA). In fact, many significant scientific breakthroughs have occurred when physicians have used prescription drugs to treat conditions outside of those formally approved uses. Many of these ''new uses'' for prescription drugs have been discovered accidentally, while others have been discovered based on the scientific and therapeutic properties of a particular prescription drug.

Prednisone is one of the best examples of applying scientific knowledge of how the drug works in the body to other potential uses. Prednisone has been used for dozens of years to treat a variety of conditions. Physicians and scientists know that the drug works in the body by decreasing the body's inflammatory and immune responses. A common problem many people will face in their lifetime is a dreaded case of poison ivy. The juice from a poison ivy plant gets on our skin, our body recognizes this as a foreign antigen or allergen, and the result is a swollen, itchy rash classified as a type of allergic reaction.

In the past, physicians knew that prednisone was effective in treating other allergic reactions, so theoretically it should be effective in treating poison ivy rash. They were correct and thus discovered a new use for prednisone. To this day, the FDA has not formally approved prednisone to treat poison ivy rash. But through medical research and the experience of millions of people who have used the drug, it is a widely accepted treatment for poison ivy. The companies who make prednisone will probably never seek formal approval for this indication because its use for poison ivy rash is so widely accepted by physicians. This example illustrates that when we know how a drug works, the knowledge can lead to other potential new uses.

Many times a new use for a drug is discovered completely by accident and is totally unrelated to how we think the drug acts in the body. A good example of this is the drug Tagamet, which has been used for years to treat acid reflux and ulcers. In fact, the drug is now available over the counter without a prescription to treat heartburn. Tagamet works primarily by blocking the receptors in the stomach that cause stomach acid to be produced. A few years ago, some physicians observed an interesting side effect of Tagamet in certain children. Some physicians noticed that a number of children who were taking large doses of Tagamet for their stomach problems for several weeks saw their skin warts heal and disappear. These observations prompted further research, and similar results were seen in some but not all children. Physicians still have no logical explanation for why Tagamet clears up warts in some children. Scientific evidence of how Prozac, Paxil, Zoloft and Luvox work in the body, as well as purely accidental discoveries through use, should help researchers to uncover other potential uses for the SSRIs as well.

As we move into the next century, expect to see Prozac, Paxil, Zoloft, and Luvox used in dozens of other types of mental illness, emotional disorders, anxiety-related disorders, and other brain chemical–related diseases. We have only begun to the scratch the surface of their potential use. In fact, three of the four drugs in this class (Zoloft, Paxil, and Luvox) have been in use only for a few years. Through research, experience, and trial and error, these drugs should gain wide acceptance for a variety of mental illness conditions in the future.

Currently, these drugs are approved only to treat major depression and obsessive-compulsive disorder (OCD). Through specialized clinical studies, Prozac has also been approved to treat bulimia nervosa, and Paxil and Zoloft have been approved to treat panic disorder. Exploratory medical research is beginning to find several other potential uses for these four drugs.

The following discussions recap the ongoing exploratory research into many new potential uses of the SSRIs. Many of these studies were conducted on small groups of patients. Other results included are presented as case studies. Case studies are reports based on physician notes from their practice and the use of these drugs in small numbers of their own patients. The results of case studies can provide valuable insight into other possible new uses of these drugs. These results, however, should be interpreted very carefully until more research is conducted in larger patient groups. *Most importantly, individuals should never use one of these drugs for any unapproved use discussed in this book without first consulting their doctor.*

SOME FUTURE USES OF PROZAC, PAXIL, ZOLOFT, AND LUVOX

Dysthymia

Dysthymia is a mild form of major depression. In general there are two types of dysthymia. The more common form is called sporadic depression. In sporadic depression, the patient has more depressed days than not, but not two continuous weeks of depression as in individuals suffering from major depression. These individuals also do not have four of the eight symptoms that characterize major depression. About 85 percent of individuals with dysthymia have sporadic depression. The other form of dysthymia is less common. These individuals have symptoms of depression every day, but they are milder than in those with major depression. These individuals also typically experience only four of the eight symptoms that characterize major depression.

Several studies have shown that SSRIs can be effective in treating dysthymia.[5–10] In one small study, patients took 20mg to 60mg of Prozac per day for approximately twelve weeks. The study found that six of the nine patients on Prozac saw an improvement in their dysthymia symptoms.[11] In another study, sixteen patients were given Prozac and sixteen patients were given a placebo (inert pill). Patients taking Prozac were given 20mg every other day or up to 60mg once daily. This study found that ten of the sixteen patients treated with Prozac saw a significant improvement in their symptoms compared to only two of the sixteen patients taking a placebo.[12] Finally, in a third study, fifty-two patients were given 20mg to 60mg of Prozac per day for six weeks. Of these patients, 73 percent observed an improvement in their symptoms.[13] Other clinical studies have shown similar results in the effectiveness of Prozac to treat dysthymia. However, more research needs to be conducted on larger numbers of patients to determine the true effectiveness of SSRIs in treating dysthymia.

Bulimia

Currently, it is not known how depression and eating disorders are related. It can be said, however, that many individuals who suffer from bulimia also suffer from depression. Prozac is already formally approved for use in treating bulimia. For specific information on Prozac's use in bulimia, see Chapter 5, "Prozac," the sections on approved uses and clinical studies. Luvox has also been investigated for its potential to treat bulimia. One small study of twenty patients found that 50mg to 150mg of Luvox per day significantly improved the symptoms of binge eating in these patients.[14] In another study, thirty-four patients took 50mg to 300mg of Luvox per day and thirty-four patients were given a placebo for nine weeks. The results showed that 75 percent of the patients taking Luvox saw a reduction in binge eating compared with only 45 percent in the placebo group.[15] Other reports from physicians' case studies show that Zoloft may also be somewhat effective in treating bulimia. However, researchers have cautioned that the true long-term benefits of SSRIs are not completely understood. Patients may relapse once treatment is stopped. Other research suggests that the higher the dose of an SSRI, the greater the reduction in binge eating, but these doses do not necessarily cause a reduction of vomiting.[16]

Anorexia Nervosa

There is limited research regarding the effectiveness of SSRIs in treating anorexia nervosa. In fact, weight loss is a side effect in some patients taking SSRIs, which is undesirable in these patients. A recent study, conducted at the University of Pittsburgh Medical Center and presented at the 1997 American Psychiatric Association's annual meeting, showed that Prozac may be effective in treating anorexia nervosa. The study found that Prozac helped patients with anorexia nervosa maintain a healthy body weight once they had regained significant amounts of weight. This study is the first of its kind to suggest that an antidepressant may prevent a relapse of anorexia nervosa. A few other case studies have also indicated some success in treating anorexia nervosa with Prozac. The true effect of SSRIs in treating this condition, however, still remains very unclear.

Weight Loss

Of all the research into other uses of SSRIs, much of it has been focused on the ability of these drugs to cause weight loss. What was once thought to be an undesirable side effect has now emerged into the potential for a large new market for these drugs. A large study was conducted on 458 patients during a one-year period. Patients taking 60mg of Prozac had significantly more weight loss than those patients taking a placebo through the first twenty-eight weeks of the study. After one year, however, no additional weight loss was seen between patients taking Prozac and those taking a placebo. Patients who were more obese tended to lose more weight.[17]

In another large study, 655 patients were given 10mg, 20mg, 40mg, or 60mg of Prozac once daily for eight weeks. The group of patients taking the highest dose (60mg per day) saw the greatest amount of weight loss compared to the patients taking the lower doses. Those patients taking higher doses did, however, report drowsiness, tiredness, and increased sweating compared to those taking lower doses.[18]

One researcher reviewed several studies of Prozac and weight loss and came to the following conclusions: Patients taking 60mg of Prozac per day saw an average weight loss of about 1.1 pounds per week. Long-term studies showed that most weight loss occurred after Prozac had been taken for twelve weeks but less than twenty weeks.[19] One study also suggested that Prozac plus behavioral therapy produced more weight loss than behavior therapy alone.[20] Finally, another study found that Prozac (average dose at 65mg per day) produced significantly more weight loss than a placebo and somewhat more weight loss than the drug Didex in 150 patients.[21]

Zoloft and Luvox also show promise in weight reduction. However, Paxil does not seem to produce the amount of weight loss seen in the other three SSRIs.

There is little doubt from the results of these studies that Prozac can cause some weight loss. However, maintaining a constant body weight once excessive weight is lost is a problem with Prozac and the other SSRIs. This is the same problem associated with other weight-loss drugs, such as Fastin, Pondimin, Adipex, Ionamin, Redux, Didrex, and the popular Fen-Phen drug combination. (Pondimin and Redux have been pulled from the market due their causing heart valve irregularities.) One small study found that of the forty-five patients taking 20–60mg Prozac lost significantly more weight than those taking a placebo but had a tendency to gain it back. In fact, after one year of treatment, there was no difference in weight loss between the Prozac group and the placebo group.[22] From this research, we see that Prozac can cause a significant amount of weight loss in the short term (up to about twenty-six weeks), but its ability to continue to produce weight loss after this time period is questionable at best. Exercise, dieting, and a change in eating habits must be used to keep the weight off after this time period.

Alcoholism
Luvox is the only SSRI that has been researched under very strict, double-blind study conditions regarding the

treatment of alcoholism. In one study of 108 patients, Luvox was found to be superior to a placebo after sixty days and ninety days of use in reducing the number of days heavy drinking occurred, percent reduction in overall alcohol consumption, and in the number of patients achieving total abstinence.[23] Certain patients saw some positive results as early as fifteen days after beginning treatment with Luvox. However, another study found that the usefulness of Luvox in treating alcoholism may be limited by the degree and severity of side effects caused by the drug.[24] Prozac has been studied in alcoholics with depression or panic disorder. One study of 188 patients found that 70 percent of the patients taking Prozac with Antabuse achieved a "good clinical" outcome regarding their alcoholism.[25] Another study was conducted with Zoloft in twenty-two alcoholics with a history of long-term drinking, multiple relapses, treatment failures, and depression. Within two weeks, 60 percent of the patients taking Zoloft reported an improvement in appetite, sleep patterns, and mood swings compared with only 25 percent of the patients taking a placebo. Within three months, 22 percent of the patients taking Zoloft reported a continued improvement in their symptoms of alcoholism.[26] It must be noted, however, that the true effect of SSRIs in treating alcoholism is still not known.

Drug Abuse
Most of the evidence regarding the effectiveness of the SSRIs in treating drug abuse is purely anecdotal. There have been some positive results in patients addicted to cocaine and opiates. These results suggest that the SSRIs may reduce cocaine consumption. However, one study found that cocaine addicts who took Prozac as well as attending counseling felt no additional effect.[27] SSRIs may be helpful in patients addicted to both cocaine and

opiates, but not in patients addicted to cocaine alone. The reasoning is that patients addicted to both cocaine and opiates tend to have higher rates of depression and thus benefit more from SSRI treatment. Another small study found that Prozac was superior to a placebo in treating heroin addicts.[28] The results of this study should, however, be interpreted very cautiously. Based on the limited amount of research available, the effectiveness of SSRIs in treating drug abuse without depression is still not known.

Social Phobia

Some positive experiences with Zoloft, Paxil, and Prozac in social phobia have been presented. One small study of twelve patients found that Zoloft was superior to a placebo in improving the symptoms of social phobia over a twelve-week period.[29] Another study found marked or moderate improvement of symptoms in fifteen of eighteen patients taking Paxil for twelve weeks.[30] Finally, other researchers have found similar results regarding Prozac's ability to treat social phobia. These results provide a good foundation for further research as to whether or not SSRIs can help patients with social phobia.

Personality Disorders

Most of the research concerning the effectiveness of SSRIs in treating personality disorders has been conducted with Prozac. One researcher conducted two studies that found that Prozac was significantly superior to a placebo in reducing the anger associated with personality disorder.[31,32] Another small study found that eight out of twelve patients with some form of personality disorder improved to a significant degree with Prozac. Many of these patients who continued taking Prozac for one to two years continued to be much or very much improved.[33] This study also found that the symptoms returned quickly if the patient stopped taking Prozac, but improvement was seen again once the patient resumed taking the drug. Finally, another small study of eleven patients taking Zoloft saw a decrease in irritability and impulsive aggression.[34] Even though the results of these studies are promising, the true effect of SSRIs in treating this condition still remains somewhat unclear.

Problematic Sexual Behaviors

A few reports and small studies have been published regarding the effectiveness of SSRIs to treat a variety of problematic sexual behaviors including paraphilia sexual addiction, exhibitionism (flashing), and cross-dressing. One small study included twenty men who had paraphilia or nonparaphilic sexual addiction. Of the twenty men treated with Prozac, sixteen saw a significant improvement in symptoms during the four-week trial.[35] Other studies have seen successful treatment regarding cross-dressing and exhibitionism.[36,37] Many of the patients who were successfully treated also had symptoms of major depression or dysthymia. This may explain why these problematic sexual behaviors improved. Also, these behaviors are similar to obsessive or compulsive-related disorders (OCD). Since the SSRIs are well known to treat OCD, it's not surprising that the problematic sexual behaviors improved as well.

Posttraumatic Stress Disorder

There have been limited studies conducted on SSRIs and their usefulness in treating posttraumatic stress disorder. In one small study, twenty-seven veterans were treated with Prozac for ten weeks. These patients started on 20mg per day and eventually increased to 80mg per day. They saw improvement after six weeks of treatment. The researchers felt that higher doses or longer durations of treatment might be required to successfully treat this condition.[38] In another small study, 24 Dutch resistance fighters from World War II were given Luvox. Researchers determined that these veterans' improvement was only modest.[39] Finally, another study of nineteen combat veterans with posttraumatic stress disorder as well as depression were given Zoloft. Twelve of the nineteen patients were much improved in many of their symptoms except insomnia.[40] These studies suggest some effectiveness of SSRIs in treating posttraumatic stress disorder, but more research is definitely needed.

Premenstrual Syndrome

Much of the experience and research in treating premenstrual syndrome (PMS) with SSRIs is with Prozac. The most powerful example of Prozac's effect in treating PMS is from a large study involving seven Canadian women's health clinics. All the patients in the study had regular menstrual cycles, were medication free, and had no medical or psychiatric illness. A total of 313 women participated in the study with 180 finishing all six parts of the study. Women taking 20mg or 60mg of Prozac observed a significant improvement in PMS-related symptoms as compared to the group that received a placebo. Women in the group taking Prozac continued to see improvement in symptoms throughout the entire study. There was no difference in improvement of symptoms between the groups that took 20mg versus 60mg. Patients taking lower doses of Prozac experienced fewer side effects than the group taking higher doses. This suggests that lower doses of Prozac are just as effective in treating PMS as higher doses and produce fewer undesirable side effects.[40,41]

Other studies have echoed the results of the study above. Two small studies, of twenty-four patients taking 20mg of Prozac, found similar improvements in PMS symptoms.[42] In another, longer-term study, sixty-four women took between 20mg and 40mg of Prozac per day for approximately nineteen months. All of the patients who continued on Prozac saw a complete or partial control of PMS symptoms.[43] These studies leave little doubt that Prozac helped control some of the symptoms of PMS in the women involved, but more research is needed.

There has been little information on the ability of other SSRIs to treat PMS until recently. A recent study of Zoloft at twelve university-affiliated out-patient psychiatry and gynecology clinics found that 62 percent of the two hundred patients who completed the study saw marked or much improvement in their PMS symptoms compared with only 32 percent of the placebo group. This suggests that Zoloft may too be useful in treating the symptoms of severe PMS. A few very small studies suggest that Paxil may be effective in treating this condition as well. This research, along with the findings of the Prozac studies, provide a good foundation for physicians to make decisions regarding the use of the SSRIs to treat PMS.

Premature Ejaculation

Both Zoloft and Paxil have been evaluated in well-controlled studies in patients who suffer from premature ejaculation. In one study, twenty-six patients were given 50mg to 200mg of Zoloft and twenty-six patients were given a placebo (inert pill). Seventeen patients in the Zoloft group reported a significant improvement in their symptoms.[44] Another study with Paxil showed similar results regarding the improvement of symptoms.[45] Finally, a small study of forty-six patients, treated with 20mg to 60mg of Prozac, reported some effectiveness in treating premature ejaculation. All of the patients in this study reported less than thirty seconds of intercourse before ejaculation prior to taking Prozac. After therapy with Prozac began, all patients reported an increase in intercourse time of at least 5 minutes or more before ejaculation.[46]

It is not surprising that the SSRIs are effective in treating many patients with premature ejaculation. Delayed or trouble ejaculating is listed as a side effect in some sexually healthy men who take one of these drugs for depression and OCD. This is a good example of an undesirable side effect in healthy men benefiting others who suffer from that condition.

Diabetic Neuropathy

Diabetic neuropathy is a painful condition that affects many diabetics. One small study compared Paxil, Tofranil, and a placebo (inert pill) in their ability to control diabetic neuropathy. Paxil and Tofranil provided significantly more pain relief than the placebo treatment. Tofranil, however, was somewhat more effective than Paxil, but more Tofranil patients dropped out of the study due to unwanted side effects. This illustrates that patients tolerated Paxil better in the study.[47]

Another study found somewhat different results. In this study, several patients were given Elavil, Norpramin, Prozac, or a placebo. In the patients taking Elavil, 74 percent saw a moderate to great relief in pain compared to 61 percent for Norpramin, 48 percent for Prozac, and 41 percent for the placebo group. The pain associated with diabetic neuropathy was improved only in depressed patients who took Prozac. This study found that Prozac was no more effective than placebo in treating the pain of diabetic neuropathy.[48] These conflicting results cast serious doubt on the usefulness of SSRIs in treating diabetic neuropathy. However, more research needs to be done.

Headache

Headache is a common side effect in some patients who take SSRIs, but some research suggests that these drugs may also help alleviate headaches. One study of thirty-eight depressed patients who suffered from chronic headaches found that 20mg per day of Prozac produced a significant relief of those headaches.[49] Another small study found similar results in patients suffering from chronic tension headaches who took Luvox.[50] A third small, exploratory study on migraine sufferers found that Prozac was somewhat more effective than a placebo.[51] Other studies, however, have not produced such dramatic results. One small study of patients suffering from chronic tension headaches found that Paxil was ineffective in treating those headaches.[52] Until more research is conducted, the questions still remains regarding the effectiveness of the SSRIs in treating various headache disorders.

Body Dysmorphic Disorder and Hypochondria

Patients suffering from both body dysmorphic disorder (BDD) and hypochondria have repetitive thoughts, behaviors, and preoccupations with the human body. In BDD, these thoughts and preoccupations concern the imagined ugliness of particular body parts or features. Patients suffering from BDD engage in repetitive mirror checking and/or have multiple surgical procedures to correct these perceived imperfections. Patients who are hypochondriacs feel that something is always wrong with their health. These patients tend to imagine different medical illnesses and make more trips than normal to the doctor to discuss these perceived illnesses. Both of these conditions are believed to be related to obsessive-compulsive disorder (OCD). Therefore, it is not surprising that some patients who have these conditions may benefit from SSRIs.

Certain case studies have found that patients with BDD responded to SSRIs, but not to tricylic antidepressants (TCAs).[53] Other researchers have found similar, positive results in small numbers of patients who have been treated with SSRIs.[54] A small study of hypochondriacs found that high doses of Prozac for twelve weeks resulted in a significant reduction in hypochondrical thoughts.[55] Other research suggests that hypochondriacs may also respond to other drugs such as Tofranil.[56] These case studies have fueled interest in conducting larger studies to examine whether or not SSRIs are truly effective in treating BDD and hypochondria. Until such research can be conducted, physicians are unsure as to how much these patients can benefit from taking SSRIs. However, these early results show some promise.

Trichotillomania

Trichotillomania (TTM) is best described as the repetitive pulling of one's own hair. Researchers believe this condition is also related to OCD. TTM most often begins during childhood and is more prevalent in females. Two studies have found that SSRIs are effective in treating TTM, but a third study found no effect. In the one study, twelve patients were given up to 80mg per day of Prozac for sixteen weeks. Researchers observed a 34 percent improvement in their TTM symptoms.[57] Most of this improvement was seen after twelve weeks of therapy with Prozac. Another study found similar results in treating TTM.[58] A third study of twenty-one TTM patients taking up to 80mg of Prozac for eighteen weeks found that Prozac had no effect.[59] This study casts some doubt on the ability of SSRIs to treat TTM until more research is done.

TEN

❧

Other New Therapies: New Drugs and St. John's Wort

As the market for prescription drugs used to treat depression and OCD continues to grow astronomically, consumers should expect to see a flood of new drugs enter the market in the future. If these drugs of the future expect to challenge Prozac, Paxil, Luvox, and Zoloft's market share, they must overcome several obstacles. They must:

1. be able to provide convenient dosing schedules.
2. have fewer side effects, adverse effects, and drug interactions.
3. demonstrate significantly greater effectiveness.
4. gain the trust of the physicians who prescribe them.

Remember that the four SSRIs are fairly new to the market themselves. Recently, a few newcomers and challengers have emerged on the antidepressant and OCD market. However, none of them has posed a formidable challenge to the SSRIs.

SERZONE

Of all the new compounds approved to treat depression, Serzone has probably enjoyed the most success. Many patients have experienced dramatic improvements in their depression while taking Serzone. This drug is becoming quite popular, but there are a few idiosyncrasies that are prohibiting the drug from achieving blockbuster status. Dr. Williams thinks that a major disadvantage of the drug is its dosing schedule. The drug has to be given twice daily. Dr. Williams believes this puts Serzone at a serious disadvantage as compared to the once-a-day dosing of Prozac, Paxil, and Luvox, because many patients want something they can take once a day.

The other problem with Serzone is the drug interaction with Hismanal. Serzone, when taken with Hismanal, can cause dangerous irregular heartbeats. Dr. Williams says, "Why take the chance when Prozac, Zoloft, Paxil, and Luvox are just as effective and don't cause that interaction?" Serzone is also known to cause more drowsiness than the SSRIs. This usually diminishes with continued use but is still a side effect many patients don't want to have to deal with. All in all, Serzone is very effective in treating depression and many patients have experienced dramatic results. These small idiosyncrasies may make the SSRIs a slightly better choice.

REMERON

This drug is more similar to the tricyclic antidepressants (TCAs) than it is to the SSRIs. This in and of itself makes it a less desirable choice. A small pharmaceutical company, Organon, markets the drug. Because Organon does not have the marketing muscle of larger pharmaceutical manufacturers, its acceptance and use among physicians may take longer. The drug needs to be taken only once per day, which makes it an attractive alternative. However, one potentially dangerous side effect has hurt the drug's appeal.

In a rare number of patients, the blood disorder known as agranulocytosis can occur. In agranulocytosis, the bone marrow is damaged and white blood cells, the body's natural defense, are not produced. This condition can be life-threatening, it but usually resolves itself once the patient stops using the drug. Many patients who take Clozaril for schizophrenia have a similar problem, according to Dr. Williams. In fact, every patient taking Clozaril must have regular blood tests. Even though this is not required for Remeron because the incidence of agranulocytosis is so rare, physicians have been cautious about prescribing Remeron.

EFFEXOR

Effexor has enjoyed some limited success upon entering the depression market. The drug was very popular when it was first introduced, but its popularity has leveled off for several reasons. Like Serzone, Effexor must be taken multiple times during the day, usually two or three times daily. This makes it harder for patients to remember to take their medication. The drug also causes a fair amount of drowsiness. Effexor is recommended to be taken with food or milk to reduce the potential for upset stomach and nausea, which may make it less convenient for some patients.

Dr. Williams does not prescribe Effexor very often for another reason as well. Effexor may raise a patient's blood pressure. Because many depressed patients either have borderline or high blood pressure, a physician is less likely to prescribe a drug that may raise blood pressure when other drugs, such as Prozac, Paxil, Luvox, and Zoloft, do not. Dr. Williams does believe, however, that the drug may be helpful in treating hyperactivity in children. This observation is based only on a small number of case studies and much more research is needed, but some results in individual children have been promising.

WELLBUTRIN SR

The drug Wellbutrin has only been available in the SR (sustained-release formulation) for a short time. The regular Wellbutrin, however, has been available for quite some time. Originally, doctors avoided Wellbutrin because of the bad press about the drug causing seizures. The drug may cause seizures in approximately 0.4 percent of patients (1 in about every 250). The risk of the drug causing a seizure is approximately four times greater for Wellbutrin than for other antidepressants. The manufacturer, however, has developed strict guidelines to help lower the risk of seizure. This potentially serious side effect, as well as having to take Wellbutrin three to four times a day, hurt the drug significantly.

Recently, the drug became available as Wellbutrin SR, which can be taken twice daily. The seizure risk is still present, but more is known about minimizing the risk of a patient having a seizure. Dr. Williams's experience is that Wellbutrin SR is a great medication and he has seen similar degrees of effectiveness in treating depression as in the SSRIs. However, a twice daily formulation like Wellbutrin SR still makes it a second choice to one of the SSRIs that may be taken once daily.

Taking your medication regularly is key to achieving improvement in your depression, according to Dr. Williams. The once daily dosing of the SSRIs makes that goal more attainable. Other physicians, however, are switching some patients from SSRIs to Wellbutrin SR in one specific circumstance. Some patients taking SSRIs experience unwanted sex-related side effects such as decreased sex drive, impotence, difficulty in having an orgasm, and so on. Wellbutrin SR seems to have a significantly lower incidence of this type of side effect.

ST. JOHN'S WORT—NATURE'S PROZAC

St. John's wort, also known as *Hypericum perforatum*, has been around for about two thousand years. Some believe that it was used in ancient Greece as a potion to drive away evil spirits. The preparation gets its name from John the Baptist. It's said that the perennial plant's bright yellow flowers are most abundant around June 24, the birthday of John the Baptist.

Historically, St. John's wort has been used as an herbal remedy for depression, anxiety, gastritis, and insomnia. It's become most popular, however, in Europe within the last fifteen years as a treatment for depression. In Germany, it's the leading treatment for depression. German physicians prescribe more than 60 million doses per year. In fact, German physicians write more prescriptions for St. John's wort than for Prozac. Even though St. John's wort has been used extensively in Europe for depression, the FDA has still not approved it for use in the United States, and it is therefore regulated as a dietary supplement. However, this may change in the future based on some new clinical studies.

St. John's wort has shown promising results in treating depression in some important clinical studies. One study compared the results of twenty-three different clinical trials involving over three thousand patients.[60] Fifteen of these studies compared St. John's wort to a placebo (inert pill) and eight studies compared it with other drugs. Overall, results of this analysis found that St. John's wort was more effective than a placebo and equally effective as some antidepressants. Also, patients taking St. John's wort experienced fewer side effects.

Another study of 105 out-patients with mild depression found similar results.[61] In this study, 67 percent of the patients taking St. John's wort saw an improvement in their symptoms compared with only 28 percent of the patients taking a placebo.

Another six-week study found that St. John's wort was as effective as the antidepressant Tofranil in reducing the symptoms associated with mild to moderate depression.[62] However, no studies have compared St. John's wort to either Prozac, Paxil, Zoloft, or Luvox.

Based on what we currently know about St. John's wort, it seems to be fairly safe to take. The compound seems to cause no adverse effects on the heart or other major organ systems when used for up to six weeks. The effect of long-term use of the compound has not been studied. Therefore, caution should be used. The drug may, however, increase the sensitivity of a patient's skin to sunlight and may cause you to sunburn more easily. Therefore, patients taking St. John's wort should use a sunscreen when outdoors.

Other side effects seem to be almost nonexistent. The most common side effects appear to be stomach upset, diarrhea, allergic reactions, and fatigue.[63] These adverse effects, however, usually affect less than 1 percent of the patients taking the compound. The usual dose is 300mg three times daily of a standardized 0.3 percent hypericin extract. The cost of a month's supply is ten to fifteen dollars.

There is, however, one important precaution that should be observed when taking St. John's wort. The drug should not be taken together with other antidepressants. This combination could cause serotonin syndrome, a potentially life-threatening condition. Serotonin syndrome is caused by having too much serotonin in the body. Never take St. John's wort with other antidepressant medications. It is also recommended that before taking St. John's wort patients should talk with their doctor or pharmacist.

References

1. Simeon, J. G., Dinicola, V. F., Ferguson, H. B., et al. (1990) Adolescent depression: a placebo-controlled fluoxetine treatment study and follow-up. *Prog Neuropsychopharmacol Biol Psychiatry* **14,** 791–795.
2. Cohen, L. S., Schneider, O., Rubin, L., et al. (1991) *Fluoxetine in Adolescent Psychiatric Inpatients.* Presented at the American Psychiatric Association Annual Meeting, New Orleans, May 11–16, 1991.
3. Rodriguez-Ramos, R., deDios Vega, J. L,, San-Sebastian-Cabases, J., et al. (1996) Effects of paroxetine in depressed adolescents. *Eur J Clin Res* (in press).
4. Jain, U., Birmaher, B., Garcia, M., et al. (1992) Fluoxetine in children and adolescents with mood disorders: A chart review of efficacy and adverse effects. *J Child Adolesc Psychopharmacol* **4,** 259–261.
5. Waring, E. M., Chamberlaine, C. H., McCrank, E. W., et al. (1988) Dysthymia: A randomized study of cognitive and marital therapy and antidepressants. *Can J Psychiatry* **33,** 96–99.
6. Kocsis, J. H. (1989) Dysthymic disorder. In: Karasu, B. (ed) *Treatment of Psychiatric Disorders,* American Psychiatric Assn., Washington, DC.
7. Dunner, D. L. and Schmaling, K. B. (1994) Treatment of dysthmia: Fluoxetine versus cognitive therapy. Pre-

sented at the XIXth Collegium Internationale Neuro-Psychopharmacologicum Congress, Washington, DC, June 27–July 1. *Neuropsychopharmacology* **10, (Number 35/Part 2),** 234S.

8. Lapierre, Y. D. (1994) Pharmacological therapy of dysthymia. *Acta Psychiatr Scand* **89 (Suppl 383),** 42–48.

9. Nobler, M. S., Devanand, D. P., Singer, T. M., et al. (1994) *Fluoxetine Treatment for Elderly Patients with Dysthymic Disorders: A Pilot Study.* Presented at the American Psychiatric Association Annual Meeting, Philadelphia, PA, May 21–26. (New Research Program and Abstracts, p 91.)

10. Ravindran, A. V., Bialik, R. J., and Lapierre, Y. D. (1994). Therapeutic efficacy of specific serotonin reuptake inhibitors (SSRIs) in dysthymia. *Can J Psychiatry* **39,** 21–26.

11. Rosenthal, J., Hemlock, C., Hellerstein, D. J., et al. (1992) A preliminary study of serotonergic antidepressants in treatment of dysthymia. *Prog Neuropsychopharmacol Biol Psychiatry* **16,** 933–941.

12. Hellerstein, D. J., Yanowitch, P., Rosenthal, J., et al. (1993) A randomized double-blind study of fluoxetine versus placebo in the treatment of dysthymia. *Am J Psychiatry* **150,** 1169–1175.

13. Ravindran, A. V., Bialik, R. J. and Lapierre, Y. D. (1994) Primary early onset dysthymia, biochemical correlates of the therapeutic response to fluoxetine: I. Platelet monoamine oxidase and the dexamethasone suppression test. *J Affect Disord* **31,** 111–117.

14. Ayuso-Gutierrez, J. L., Palazon, M. and Ayuso-Mateos, J. L. (1994) Open trial of fluvoxamine in the treatment of bulimia nervosa. *Int J Eating Disord* **15,** 245–249.

15. Gardiner, H. M., Freeman, C.P., Jesinger, D. K., et al. (1993) Fluvoxamine: An open pilot study in moderately obese female patients suffering from atypical eating disorders and episodes of bingeing. *Int J Obes* **17,** 301–305.

16. Boyer, W. and Feighner, J. P. (1994) *Antidepressant Dose-response Relationship in Bulimia.* Presented at the XIX Collegium Internationale Neuro-Psychopharmacologiucum

Meeting, Washington, DC, June 27–July 1, 1994.

17. Goldstein, D. J., Rampey, A. H. Jr., Enas, G. G., et al. (1994) Fluoxetine: A randomized clinical trial in the treatment of obesity. *Int J Obes* **18,** 129–135.

18. Levine, L. R., Enas, G. G., Thompson, W. L., et al. (1989) Use of fluoxetine, a selective serotonin-reuptake inhibitor, in the treatment of obesity: A dose-response study. *Int J Obes* **13,** 635–645.

19. Wise, S. D. (1992) Clinical studies with fluoxetine in obesity. *Am J Clin Nutr* **55,** 181S-184S.

20. Marcus, M. D., Wing, R. R., Ewing, L., et al. (1990) A double-blind, placebo-controlled trial of fluoxetine plus behavior modification in the treatment of obese binge-eaters and non-binge-eaters. *Am J Psychiatry* **147,** 876–881.

21. Ferguson, J. M. and Feighner, J. P. (1987) Fluoxetine-induced weight loss in overweight nondepressed humans. *Int J Obes* **11 (Suppl 3),** 163–170.

22. Darga, L. L., Carroll-Michals, L., Botsford, S. J., et al. (1991) Fluoxetine's effect on weight loss in obese subjects. *Am J Clin Nutr* **54,** 321–325.

23. Block, B. A., Holland, R. I., and Ades, J. (1994) *Recidivist Alcoholics: A Double-blind, Placebo-controlled Study of Fluvoxamine.* Presented at the XIX CINP Meeting, Washington, DC, 1994.

24. Kranzler, H. R., Del-Boca, F., Korner, P., et al. (1993) Adverse effects limit the usefulness of fluvoxamine for the treatment of alcoholism. *J Subst Abuse Treat* **10,** 283–287.

25. Borup, C. and Unden, M. (1994) Combined fluoxetine and disulfiram treatment of alcoholism with comorbid affective disorders. A naturalistic outcome study, including quality of life measurements. *Eur Psychiatry* **9,** 83–89.

26. O'Brien, K. (1994) *Depression Seen During Alcohol Detoxification: Early Intervention with Sertraline.* Presented at the XIX CINP Meeting, Washington, DC, 1994.

27. Covi, L., Hess, J. M., Haertzen, C. A., et al. (1992) *Fluoxetine and Counseling in Cocaine Abuse.* Presented at the

American Psychiatric Association Annual Meeting, Washington, DC, May 2–7, 1992.

28. Gerra, G., Fertonani, G., Zaimovic, A., et al. (1994) *Hostility in Substance Abusers Subtypes: Fluoxetine and Naltrexone Treatment.* Presented at the XIX CINP Meeting, Washington, DC, 1994.

29. Katzelnick, D. J., Greist, J. H., Jefferson, J. W., et al. (1994) *Sertraline in Social Phobia: A Controlled Pilot Study.* Presented at the XIX CINP Meeting, Washington, DC, May 20–25, 1994.

30. Mancini, C. L. (1995) *An Open Trial of Paroxetine in Social Phobia.* Presented at the American Psychiatric Association Annual Meeting, Miami, FL, 1995.

31. Salzman, C. (1994) *Effect of Fluoxetine on Anger in Borderline Personality Disorder.* Presented at the XIX CINP Meeting, Washington, DC, 1994.

32. Salzman, C., Schatzberg, A.F., Miyawaki, E., et al. (1992) *Fluoxetine in BPD.* Presented at the American Psychiatric Association Annual Meeting, Washington, DC, May 2–7, 1992.

33. Norden, M. J. (1989) Fluoxetine in borderline personality disorder. *Prog Neuropsychopharmacol Biol Psychiatry* **13,** 885–893.

34. Kavoussi, R. J., Liu, J., and Coccaro, E. F. (1994) An open trial of sertraline in personality disordered patients with impulsive aggression. *J Clin Psychiatry* **55,** 137–141.

35. Kafka, M. P. and Prentky, R. (1992) Fluoxetine treatment of nonparaphilic sexual addictions and paraphilias in men. *J Clin Psychiatry* **53,** 351–358.

36. Kafka, M. P. (1991) Successful treatment of paraphilic coercive disorder (a rapist) with fluoxetine hydrochloride. *Br J Psychiatry* **158,** 844–847.

37. Jorgensen, J. T. (1990) Cross-dressing successfully treated with fluoxetine. *NY State J Med* **90,** 566–567.

38. Nagy, L. M., Morgan, C. A., Southwick, S. M., et al. (1993) Open prospective trial of fluoxetine for posttraumatic stress disorder. *J Clin Psychopharmacol* **13,** 107–113.

39. Den Boer, M., Op-den-Velde, W., Falger, P. J., et al.

(1992) Fluvoxamine treatment for chronic PTSD: A pilot study. *Psychother Psychosom* **57,** 158–163.

40. Kline, N. A., Dow, B. M., Brown, S. A. et al. (1993) Sertraline for Posttraumatic Stress Disorder with Comorbid Major Depression. Presented at the American Psychiatric Association Annual Meeting, San Francisco, CA, May 22–27.

41. Menkes, D. B., Taghavi, E., Mason, P. A., et al. (1993) Fluoxetine's spectrum of action in premenstrual syndrome. *Int Clin Psychopharmacol* **8,** 95–102.

42. Steiner, M., Oakes, R., Gergel, I. P., et al. (1995) *A Fixed Dose Study of Paroxetine and Placebo in the Treatment of Panic Disorder.* Presented at the American Psychiatric Association Annual Meeting, Miami, FL, May 20–25, 1995.

43. Wood, S. H., Mortola, J. F., Chan, Y. F., et al. (1992) Treatment of premenstrual syndrome with fluoxetine: a double-blind, placebo-controlled, crossover study. *Obstet Gynecol* **80 (3 Pt 1),** 339–344.

44. Pearlstein, T. B., Stone, A. B. (1994) Long-term treatment of late luteal phase dysphoric disorder. *J Clin Psychiatry* **55 (8, Aug),** 332–335.

45. Meudels, J., Camera, A. (1994) Sertraline treatment for premature ejaculation. Presented at the XIX CINP meeting, Washington, DC, 1994.

46. Waldinger, M. D., Hengeveld, M. W., and Zwinderman, A. H. (1994) Paroxetine treatment of premature ejaculation: a double-blind, placebo-controlled study. *Am J Psychiatry* **151,** 1377–1379.

47. Crenshaw, R. T. and Wiesner, M. G. (1992) *Treatment of Premature Ejaculation with Prozac.* Presented at the American Psychiatric Association Annual Meeting, Washington, DC, 1992.

48. Sindrup, S. H., Gram, L. F., Brsen, K., et al. (1990) The selective serotonin reuptake inhibitor paroxetine is effective in the treatment of diabetic neuropathy symptoms. *Pain* **42,** 135–144.

49. Max, M. B., Lynch, S. A., Muir, J., et al. (1992) Effects of desipramine, amitriptyline, and fluoxetine on pain in

diabetic neuropathy. *N Engl J Med* **326,** 1250–1256.

50. Diamond, S. and Freitag, F. G. (1989) The use of fluoxetine in the treatment of headache. *Clin J Pain* **5,** 200–201.

51. Manna, V., Bolino, F., and Di-Cicco, L. (1994) Chronic tension-type headache, mood depression and serotonin: therapeutic effects of fluvoxamine and mianserine. *Headache* **34,** 44–49.

52. Adly, C., Straumanis, J., and Chesson, A. (1992) Fluoxetine prophylaxis of migraine. *Headache* **32,** 101–104.

53. Langemark, M. and Olesen, J. (1994) Sulpiride and paroxetine in the treatment of chronic tension-type headache. An explanatory double-blind trial. *Headache* **34,** 20–24.

54. Hollander, E., Liebowitz, M. R., Winchel, R., et al. (1990) Treatment of body dysmorphic disorder with serotonin reuptake blockers. *Am J Psychiatry* **146,** 768–770.

55. Phillips, K. S., McElroy, S. I., Keck, P. E. Jr,, et al. (1993) Body dysmorphic disorder: 30 cases of imagined ugliness. *Am J Psychiatry* **150,** 302–308.

56. Fallon, B. A., Liebowitz, M. R., Salman, E., et al. (1993) Fluoxetine for hypochondriacal patients without major depression. *J Clin Psychopharmacol* **13,** 438–441.

57. Wesner, R. B. and Noyes, R. (1991) Imipramine an effective treatment for illness phobia. *J Affect Disord* **22,** 43–48.

58. Winchel, R. M., Jones, J. S., Stanley, B., et al. (1992) Clinical characteristics of trichotillomania and its response to fluoxetine. *J Clin Psychiatry* **53,** 304–308.

59. Koran, L. M., Ringold, A. and Hewlett, W. (1992) Fluoxetine for trichotillomania: An open clinical trial. *Psychopharmacol Bull* **28,** 145–149.

60. Christenson, G. A., Mackenzie, T. B., Mitchell, J. E., et al. (1991) A placebo-controlled, double-blind, crossover study of fluoxetine in trichotillomania. *Am J Psychiatry* **148,** 1566–1571.

61. Linde, K. et al. (1996) St. John's Wort for depression— an overview and meta-analysis of randomized clinical trials. *British Medical Journal* **313**: 253–258.

62. Sommer, H. et al. (1994) Placebo-controlled double-blind study examining the effectiveness of hypericum preparation in 105 mildly depressed patients. *Journal of Geriatr Psychiatry Neurol* **7: (supplement 1)** S9–11.

63. Vorbach, E. U. et al. (1994) Effectiveness and tolerance of hypericum extract LI 160 in comparison with imipramine: randomized double-blind study with 135 outpatients. *Journal of Geriatr Psychiatry Neurol* **7**: (supplement 1) S19–23.

Index

Complete and Authoritative
Health Care Books From Avon

MAKE YOUR MEDICINE SAFE
**How to Prevent Side Effects
from the Drugs You Take** by Jay Sylvan Cohen, M.D.
79075-0/$7.50 US/$9.50 Can

ST. JOHN'S WORT: NATURE'S
MOOD BOOSTER by Michael E. Thase, M.D.
Everything You Need & Elizabeth E. Loredo
to Know About This Natural Antidepressant
80288-0/$5.99 US/$7.99 Can

THE OSTEOPOROSIS CURE
**Reverse the Crippling Effects
with New Treatments** by Harris McIlwain, M.D.
79336-9/$5.99 US/$7.99 Can and Debra Fulghum Bruce

MIGRANES: **Everything You Need to Know
About Their Cause and Cure**
79077-7/$5.99 US/$7.99 Can by Arthur Elkind, M.D.

ESTROGEN: **Answers to All Your Questions**
79076-9/$5.99 US/$7.99 Can by Mark Stolar, M.D.

A HANDBOOK OF NATURAL
FOLK REMEDIES by Elena Oumano, Ph.D.
78448-3/$5.99 US/$7.99 Can

Expertly detailed, pharmaceutical guides
can now be at your fingertips
from U.S. Pharmacopeia

THE USP GUIDE TO MEDICINES
78092-5/$6.99 US/$8.99 Can

- More than 2,000 entries for both prescription and non-prescription drugs
- Handsomely detailed color insert

THE USP GUIDE TO HEART MEDICINES
78094-1/$6.99 US/$8.99 Can

- Side effects and proper dosages for over 400 brand-name and generic drugs
- Breakdown of heart ailments such as angina, high cholesterol and high blood pressure

THE USP GUIDE TO VITAMINS AND MINERALS
78093-3/$6.99 US/$8.99 Can

- Precautions for children, senior citizens and pregnant women
- Latest findings and benefits of dietary supplements

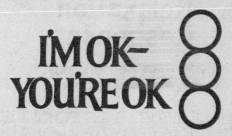

THE NATIONWIDE #1 BESTSELLER

the Relaxation Response

by Herbert Benson, M.D.
with Miriam Z. Klipper

A SIMPLE MEDITATIVE TECHNIQUE THAT HAS HELPED MILLIONS TO COPE WITH FATIGUE, ANXIETY AND STRESS

Available Now—
00676-6/ $6.99 US/ $8.99 Can